Walid Feki
Rim Kammoun
Hamdi Moalla

Smoking among medical residents

Walid Feki
Rim Kammoun
Hamdi Moalla

Smoking among medical residents

Habits, knowledge and withdrawal assistance

ScienciaScripts

Imprint
Any brand names and product names mentioned in this book are subject to trademark, brand or patent protection and are trademarks or registered trademarks of their respective holders. The use of brand names, product names, common names, trade names, product descriptions etc. even without a particular marking in this work is in no way to be construed to mean that such names may be regarded as unrestricted in respect of trademark and brand protection legislation and could thus be used by anyone.

Cover image: www.ingimage.com

This book is a translation from the original published under ISBN 978-620-6-71348-7.

Publisher:
Sciencia Scripts
is a trademark of
Dodo Books Indian Ocean Ltd. and OmniScriptum S.R.L publishing group

120 High Road, East Finchley, London, N2 9ED, United Kingdom
Str. Armeneasca 28/1, office 1, Chisinau MD-2012, Republic of Moldova, Europe
Printed at: see last page
ISBN: 978-620-7-66370-5

PLAN

INTRODUCTION

Smoking is currently a major public health problem in Tunisia and throughout the world, and is responsible for a fairly high morbidity and mortality rate **[1].** According to the World Health Organisation (WHO), 5.4 million people die from smoking every year **[2].**

This rate is rising steadily, particularly in developing countries. In fact, the WHO report on the global tobacco epidemic in 2017 showed that 11.4% of young Tunisians aged between 13 and 15 are smokers.**[3]** and that 24.9% of Tunisian adults are smokers **[4].** This scourge is currently affecting younger and younger people **[5].**

Efforts should therefore be made at all levels to control the smoking epidemic in our country. In the fight against smoking, it has been well established that to reduce smoking, healthcare professionals (HCPs) must be at the forefront and that their role is critical [**6].** The code of practice adopted by the WHO in 2004 encourages HCPs to set an example by not smoking and to play an active part in the fight against smoking **[7].**

As a result, all healthcare professionals are concerned, and have a duty to warn their patients of the many risks involved in smoking. They must make every effort to help their patients stop smoking.So they must be the first to set a good example, not to smoke and to play an active part in the fight against smoking. In this context, minimal advice on quitting smoking is an essential part of smoking prevention. Minimal advice on smoking cessation is a brief, systematic intervention that any doctor can provide when in the presence of a smoker during a consultation.Advising patients to stop smoking is an important task for all hospital staff **[8]. It is** therefore difficult to create an environment conducive to a healthy lifestyle without involving hospital staff and withouthelp the smokers among them to quit their habit. All health professionals have a role to play in this area, and must set an example to avoid any lack of effectiveness or discredit among smokers.Medical residents are key contacts for patients and therefore have an essential role to play in smoking prevention. They have a key role to play in this fight by helping to reduce smoking and its harmful effects.

Medical residents must include the fight against smoking as an integral part of their activities. In this context, the aim of our study of medical residents in Sfax is to determine the prevalence of smoking in this professional category, to assess their behaviour and attitudes towards smoking, and to assess their role in the fight against smoking.

SUBJECTS AND METHODS

1. Type of study

This is a cross-sectional study.

2. Study period

Data was collected over a 2-month period from 1er February 2016 to 31 March 2016.

3. Study population

The study population consisted of residents of the Hedi Chaker and Habib Bourguiba university hospital centres (CHU) in Sfax, meeting the following criteria:

3.1. Inclusion criteria

- Medical residents, whatever their speciality: medical, surgical or basic sciences.
- Operating during the first six months of 2016

3.2. Non-inclusion criteria

- Specialist doctors: assistants, associate professors and university hospital professors.
- Medical interns and externs.

3.3. Exclusion criteria

- Residents who gave partial replies to the questionnaire

4. Breakdown

The study subjects were divided into three groups:

- Group I: smokers are those who smoke a tobacco product at least once a day.

- Group II: Ex-smokers are those who have already smoked and do not want to smoke. smoked more than 2 years longer than when the study was carried out.

- Group III: Non-smokers are those who have never smoked.

5. Data collection

5.1. Questionnaire

The study was carried out in the form of a questionnaire drafted in French **(Appendix 1)**. The questionnaire consisted of two types of questions: closed questions where the choice of answer was imposed from a list of proposals, and open questions where the practitioner was free to propose an answer. The questionnaire was divided into four parts:

. A common area

. A section for smokers

. A game for ex-smokers

. A section for non-smokers

5.1.1. Common area

The initial part of the questionnaire was common to all the forms.

This is an information section with ten questions on :

- The doctor's civil status (nationality, age, sex, marital status, place of residence prior to medical studies)
- Professional activity (year of residency, speciality, number of hours worked per day, number of shifts per month)
- Smoking status (smoker, ex-smoker, non-smoker)

5.1.2. For smokers

The second part consisted of 44 questions of interest to residents who smoke:

- Two questions about the form and type of tobacco.
- Three questions about the age at which people start smoking and their level of education.
- A question about smoking in the family.

- A question about the number of cigarettes per day.
- Two questions about the timing of smoking.
- Four questions about smoking conditions.
- Two questions on the key causes of smoking.
- A question about the substances used.
- Four questions on the relationship between smoking and academic and professional careers.
- A question about patient advice.
- Four questions on the chances of quitting smoking and the future of smoking.
- Eight questions about the desire to stop and the means used.
- Three questions on tobacco prices and treatment reimbursement
- A question about smoking-related illnesses.
- Three questions about the doctor-patient relationship in the context of smoking.
- Three questions on smoking bans and advertising.
- A question assessing the number of doctors motivated by the possibility of further training on the subject.

5.1.3. Part for ex-smokers

The third part included 23 questions of interest to ex-smoking residents

- A question about continuing to smoke before giving up.
- A question on smoking status before 6 months.
- Two questions about the age at which people start and stop smoking.
- A question about the number of cigarettes smoked per day.
- A question about the main smoking location.
- A question about the causes of smoking.
- Two questions on the number of attempts t o stop smoking and the

treatments used to stop smoking.

- Two questions on the influence of medical studies on the quantity of cigarettes smoked.
- A question about why people stop smoking.
- A question about the desire to smoke again.
- A question about smoking in the family.
- A question about smoking-related illnesses.
- Four questions about the doctor-patient relationship in the context of smoking.
- Three questions on smoking bans and advertising.
- A question assessing the number of doctors motivated by the possibility of further training on the subject.

5.1.4. Non-smokers' section

The fourth part consisted of 14 questions of interest to non-smoking residents:

- A question about the tobacco trial.
- A question about smoking in the family.
- A question about the desire to smoke.
- A question about the places most exposed to smoking.
- A question about smoking-related illnesses.
- Three questions about the doctor-patient relationship in the context of smoking.
- Three questions on smoking bans and advertising.
- A question assessing doctors' motivation for further training on the subject.
- Two questions on the factors that encourage doctors to smoke and the possible causes of smoking cessation.

5.2. Contact with doctors

5.2.1. The first stage

The residents of the various departments were informed that they would be carrying out a survey on a topical medical subject (although the subject was kept secret from them to avoid bias) as part of a medical thesis. Residents were then given the opportunity to agree or refuse to participate. Those who were absent on the day of the information session were considered to have refused to take part. Residents who agreed to participate indicated the most suitable days to receive the questionnaire.

5.2.2. The second stage

The second contact concerned the residents who had agreed to participate. The time was chosen according to the availability of the medical team in each department, i.e. outside on-call, consultation or operating theatre hours. The interviewer delivered the questionnaire personally to each resident.

5.2.3. The third stage

The third stage consisted of recovering the various completed copies after two days. Copies that had not been completed were not considered invalid. A second request to answer the questionnaire was made.

5.2.4. The fourth beat

The fourth stage consisted of recovering all the copies after 4 days of the first recovery. Copies not completed during this second recovery were considered invalid and thus excluded from the survey.

6. Statistical study

Data from the complete forms were entered and analysed using SPSS II version 20.0 software. Incompletely completed forms were discarded. Numerical values were expressed as mean plus or minus standard deviation. The association between qualitative variables was calculated using Fisher's corrected Chi2 test for small numbers. Comparisons between quantitative variables were made using Student's T test. Significance is acquired for a $p < 0.05$ for all statistical tests.

RESULTS

1. Analysis of participation

1.1.Participation rate

The total number of residents in the Sfax university hospitals during the study period was 285. Of these, 277 agreed to take part in the survey. Of these, 222 answered the questionnaire correctly, giving an overall participation rate of 78%.

1.2.Non-respondents

Residents who did not respond to the questionnaire can be divided into two categories:
1.1.1. Those who declined to take part in the study when first approached (8 residents).

The reasons given were :

- Too many requests and not enough time to answer the questionnaires (5 residents).
- Lack of interest in surveys (1 resident)
- No reason (2 residents)

1.1.2. Those who initially agreed to respond but who were not present on the day the questionnaires were distributed (48 residents).
1.1.3. Those who responded but whose forms were incomplete and therefore unusable (7 residents).

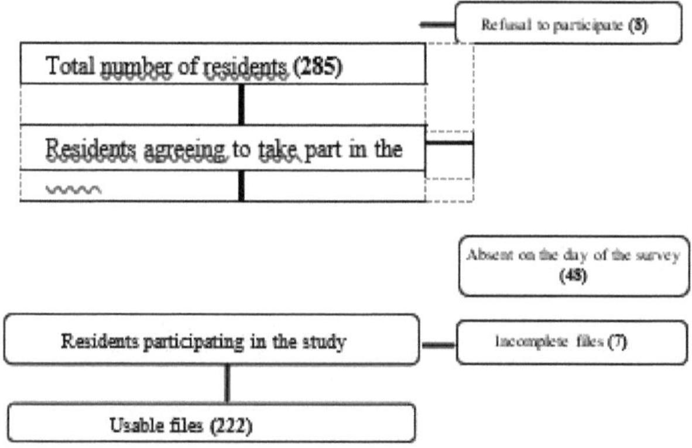

Figure 1: Analysis of residents' participation in the questionnaire.

2. Features of the population of residents who answered the questionnaire correctly

2.1. Socio-demographic characteristics

2.1.1. Age :

The average age ofthe residents included in the study was 28.38 years, with extremes ranging from 25 to 34 years.

The two most represented age groups were [27-28] and [28-29].

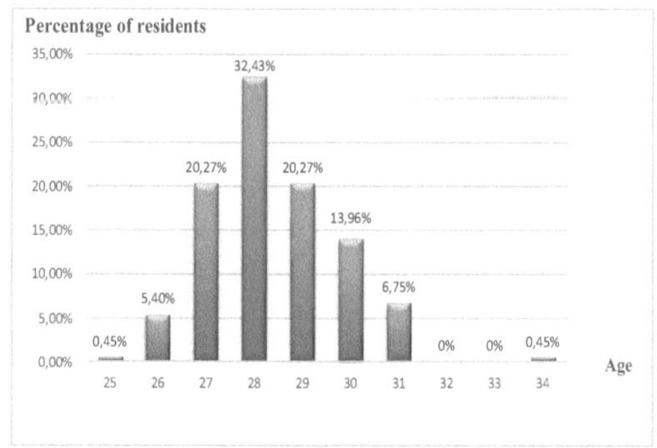

Figure 2: Breakdown of residents surveyed by age.

2.1.2. Gender

The highest percentage of residents surveyed was female (52.70 %).

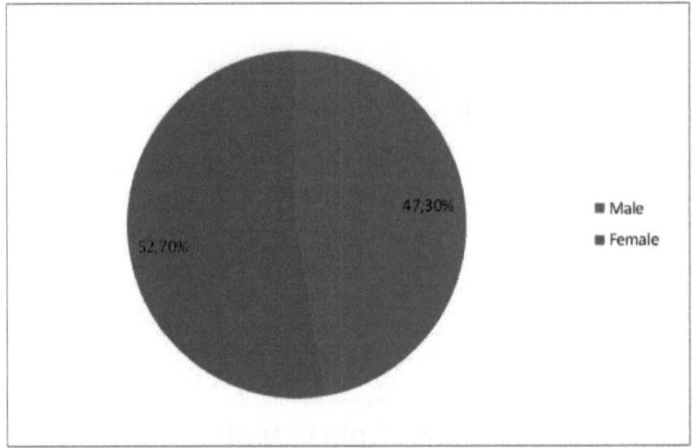

Figure 3: Breakdown of participating residents by gender.

2.1.3. Marital status

Half of the residents were married at the time of the survey (52.7%). The married residents were distributed as follows: 20 smokers, 1 ex-smoker, 96 non-smokers.

Table I: Breakdown of residents by status.

	Workforce	Percentage (%)
Married	117	52,7
Single	105	47,3

2.2.Medical studies

2.2.1. Home before medical studies

The majority of residents surveyed lived in Sfax (92.8%).

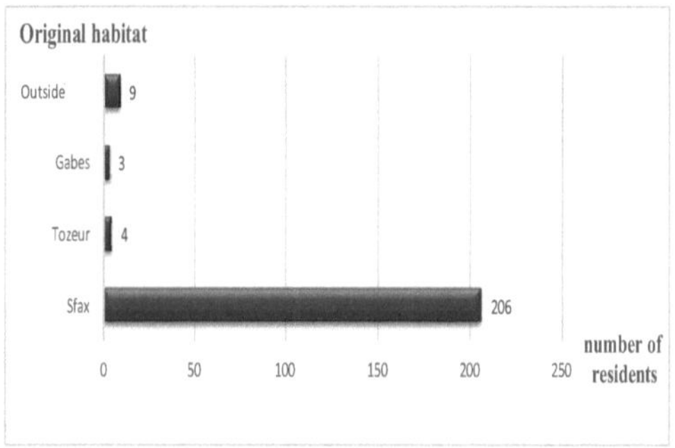

Figure 4: Distribution of residents surveyed according to their place of origin.

2.2.2. Level of study

The residents' year of study varied between 1st year and 5th year. The majority were in 2nd year.

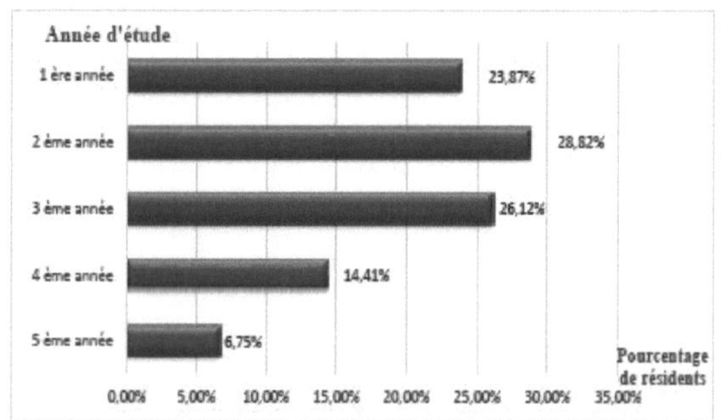

Figure 5: Breakdown of residents surveyed by year of study.

2.2.3. Specialities

The participating residents had medical (123 residents), surgical (60 residents) and basic (36 residents) specialities. Details of the specialities are shown in the table below.

Table II: Distribution of residents according to their specialities.

Specialities	Number of residents	Number of respondents	Response rate as a percentage
Fundamentals			
Biology	38	31	81.57
Genetics	2	2	100
Anatomopathology	6	3	50
Total	46	36	78
Medical			
Pneumology	6	6	100
Anaesthesia resuscitation	19	10	52.6
Neurology	7	6	85
Psychiatry	15	13	86
Nuclear medicine	1	1	100
Gastrology	1	1	100
Occupational Medicine	3	3	100
Resuscitation medical	8	6	75
Internal medicine	3	2	66
Carcinology medical	6	5	83
Rheumatology	2	1	50
Infectious	7	7	100
Physical medicine	3	3	100
Dermatology	4	4	100
Haematology	3	3	100
Paediatrics	24	17	70.8
Forensic medicine	3	2	66
Radiology	16	12	75
Preventive medicine	1	1	100
Internal medicine	3	2	66
Cardiology	7	7	100
Endocrinology	4	3	75
Nephrology	4	4	100
Radiotherapy	1	1	100

SAMU	9	6	66
Total	160	126	78.75
Surgical			
Maxillofacial	4	3	75
ENT	7	7	100
Orthopaedics	10	10	100
Cardiovascular and thoracic	6	6	100
Urology	6	3	50
Gynaecology obstetrics	15	14	93
Ophthalmology	8	3	37
Paediatric surgery	4	3	75
Neurosurgery	6	4	66
General surgery	13	7	53
Total	79	60	76
Total	285	222	78

3. Smoking status of residents

The residents included in our study were classified as "non-smokers" and "non-smokers"."The results of the survey were then compared with those of the 'smokers' survey based on the criteria set out in the methodology. The group of ex-smokers was included in the group of non-smokers because they had been smoking for 02 years or more.

3.1.Prevalence of smoking among residents

The prevalence of smoking among residents was 32.88%.

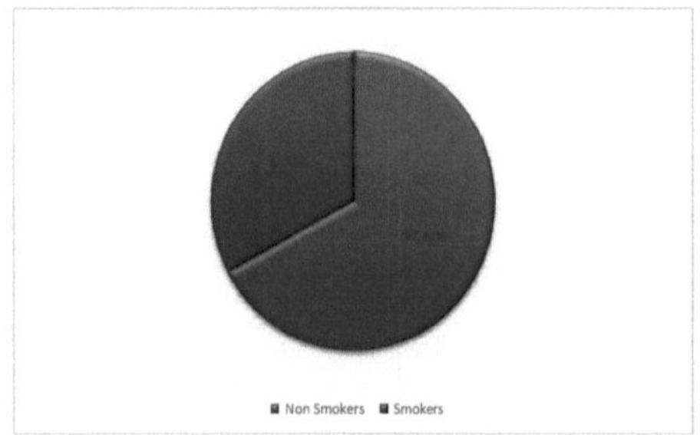

Figure 6: Prevalence of smoking among residents.

3.2. Smoking prevalence by sex

The group of smokers was represented by 73 residents, 97.26% of whom were male. The breakdown in relation to the total number is shown in the graph below:

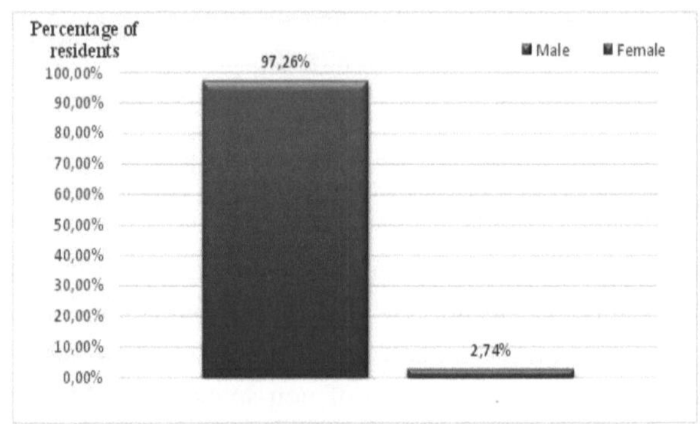

Figure 7: Prevalence of smoking by sex.

3.3. Smoking prevalence by age

The age group most affected is between 27 and 29.

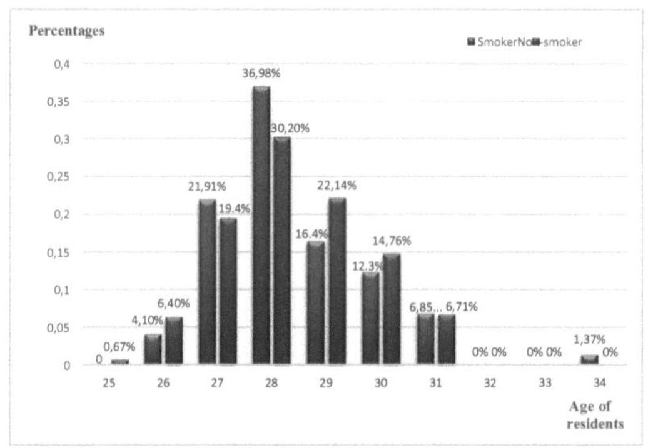

Figure 8: Prevalence of smoking by age.

3.4.Prevalence of smoking by marital status

We note that 51% of single people were smokers and only 17% of married people were smokers.

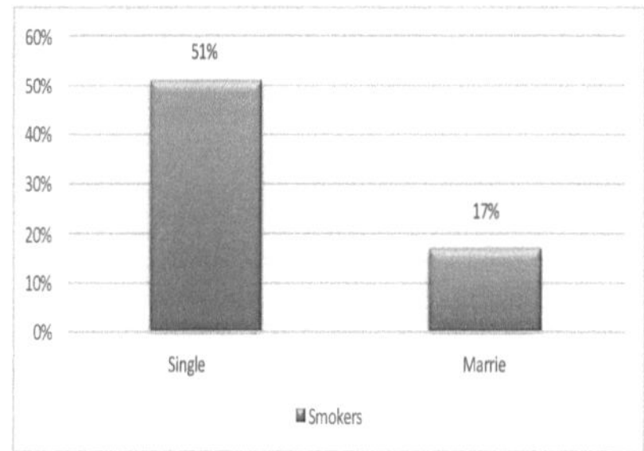

Figure 9: Prevalence of smoking by marital status.

3.5. Prevalence of smoking by specialty

The majority of residents who smoked were in surgical specialties, with a prevalence of 73.33%. This is represented in the following graph:

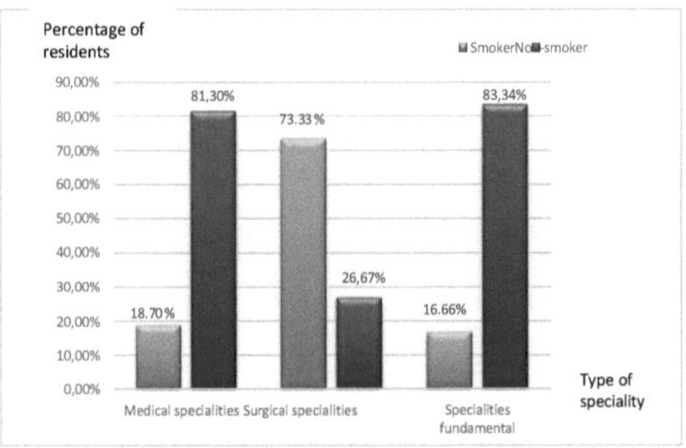

Figure 10: Percentage of smokers compared with residents in the specialty group.

3.6. Prevalence of smoking by level of education

The number of smokers was lower among residents at the end of their speciality (4^{ème}year and 5ème year).The number of smokers was highest in the first two years of specialisation.

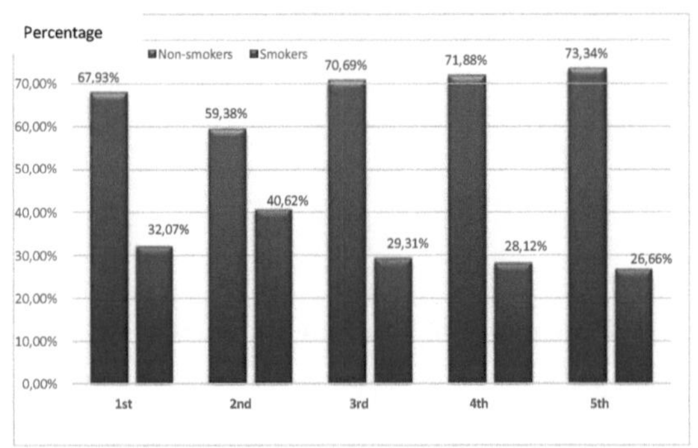

Figure 11: Prevalence of smoking by level of education.

3.7. Smoking prevalence by number of hours worked per day

Outside on-call duty, smokers worked less than non-smokers, with a statistically insignificant difference: $p = 0.87$.

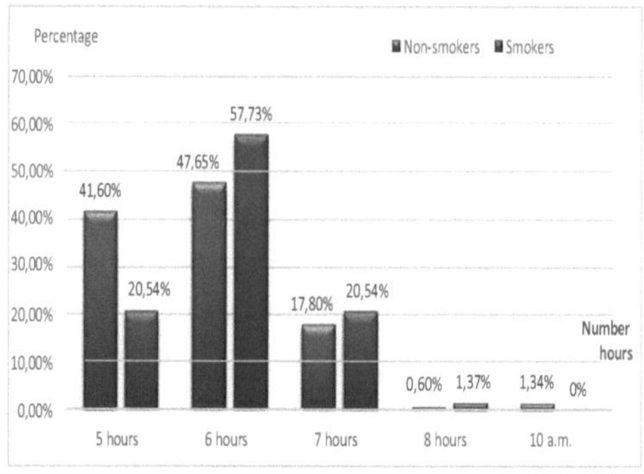

Figure 12: Prevalence of smoking by number of hours worked per day.

3.8. Prevalence of smoking by number of shifts per month

The majority of residents were on call. The average number of shifts per month for smokers was 7, higher than for non-smokers who had an average of 4 to 6 shifts, with a statistically significant difference: p = 0. The distribution of the number of shifts according to smoking status was as follows:

Table III: Prevalence of smoking according to the number of shifts per month.

Number of shifts per month	Smokers	Percentage of smokers (%)	Non-Smokers	Percentage compared with non-smoking group (%)
0	3	4.1	26	17.44
[1-3]	5	6.8	22	14.76
[4-6]	23	31.5	76	51
7	33	45.2	16	10.73
[8-9]	8	10.95	6	4
[10-12]	1	1.36	3	2

4. Characteristics of smoking among smokers

4.1.Factors influencing smoking

The average age of smoking initiation was 22 years, with extremes ranging from 12 to 25 years. Several factors were assessed to determine their influence on smoking initiation.

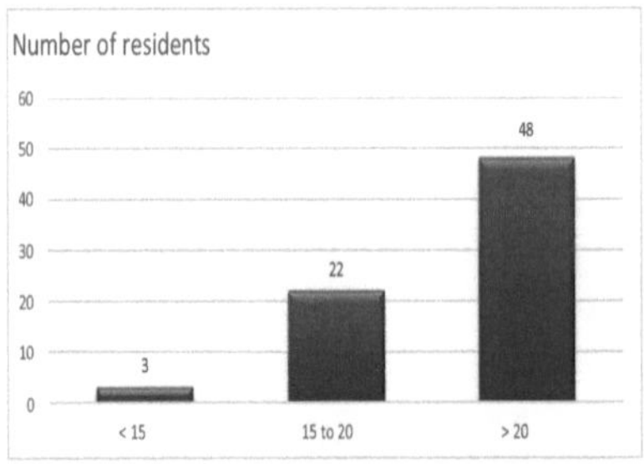

Figure 13: Age of 1st cigarette.

4.1.1. Influence of geographical origin before medical studies

There was a statistically insignificant difference between the two groups, smokers and non-smokers: $p > 0.05$. The breakdown of geographical origin before medical studies was as follows:

Table IV: Influence of geographical origin prior to medical studies.

Smoking status	Sfax	Tozeur	Gabes	Outside Tunisia	Total
Smoker	65	4	3	1	73
Non-smoking	141	0	0	8	149
Total	206	4	3	9	222

4.1.2. Influence of family and friends smoking

The circle of residents who smoked included smokers who varied between father, mother, brother and partner. All the residents surveyed had smokers in their circle (irrespective of smoking status or sex), with no statistically significant difference).

Table V: Smoking by family and friends.

	Smoker	Non-Smoking	Total
Father	44	0	44
Mother	2	0	2
Brother	27	25	52
Companion	3	121	124
Total	76	146	222

4.1.3 Influence of medical studies

4.1.3.1 Influence of the clerkship exam period

Fifty-eight residents were influenced by the clerkship period. The clerkship examination period increased the amount smoked by 79.45% of all residents who smoked.

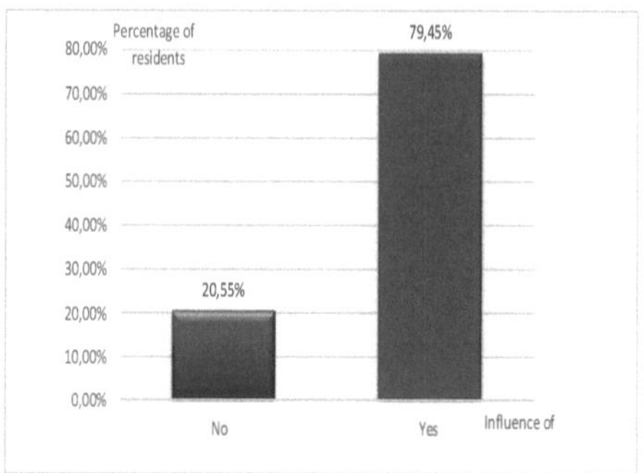

Figure 14: Influence of clerkship exam period on smoking.

4.1.3.2 Influence of the internship period

The majority of residents reported an increase in smoking at the time of their internship. Only 1.44% reported a decrease in smoking during this period.

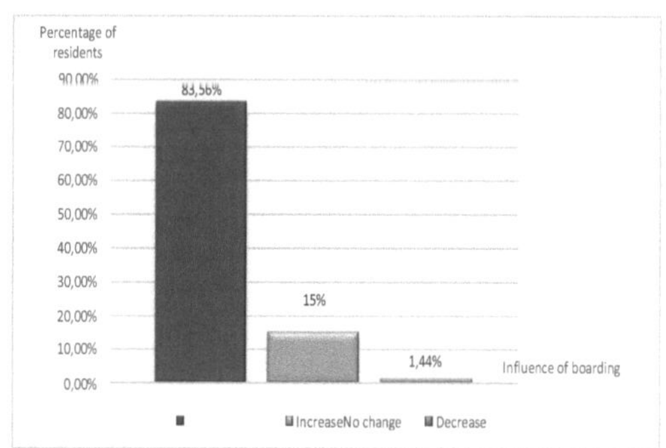

Figure 15: Influence of boarding period on tobacco consumption.

4.1.3.3 Influence of the residency competition

Passing the residency competition had a statistically significant influence on residents' smoking habits.

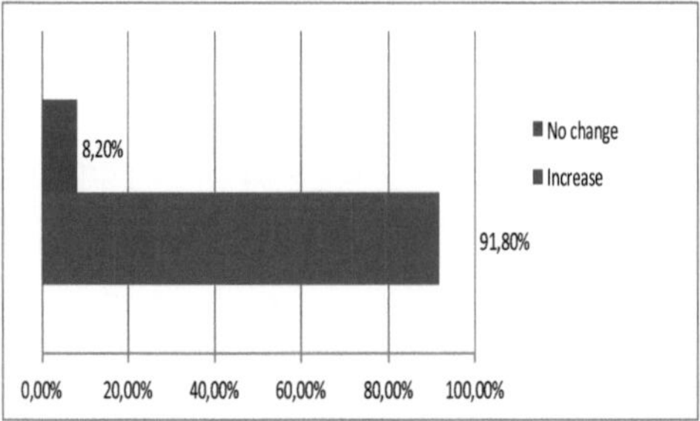

Figure 16: Influence of preparation for the residency competition on the amount smoked by residents.

4.1.4 Influence of cigarette prices

To the question "Has your tobacco consumption been influenced by the increase in the price of tobacco?", 97.3% of residents answered "no".

4.2. Smoking initiation

4.2.1. Age of smoking

The average age at which regular smoking began was 22, with extremes ranging from 14 to 25.

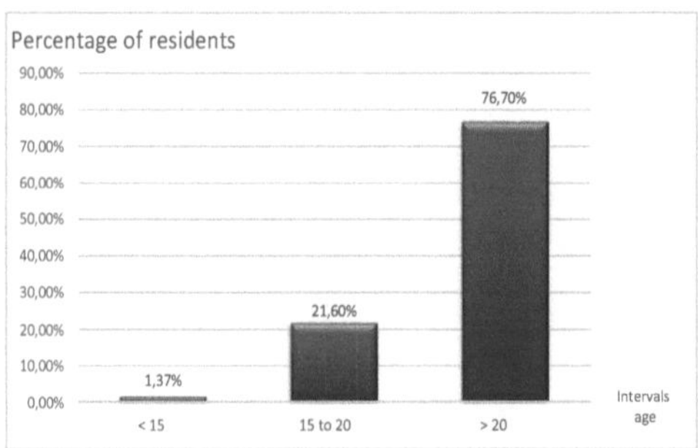

Figure 17: Age of onset of regular smoking.

4.2.2. Predictors of smoking initiation

Several factors were evaluated as predictors of smoking initiation. The most frequently cited was stress (49.3%), followed by pleasure (19.2%).

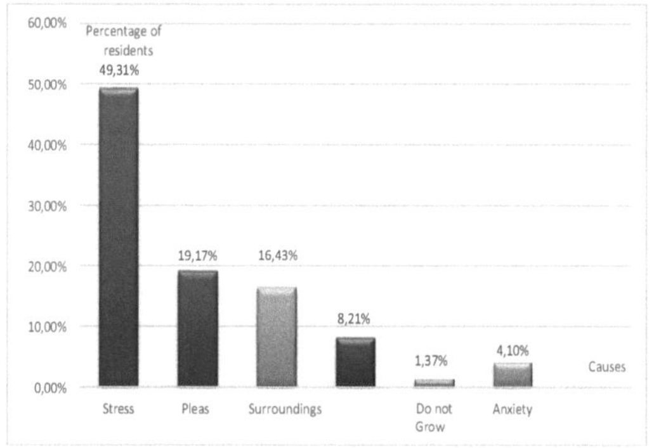

Figure 18: Causes of smoking initiation.

4.2.3. Factors predictive of continued smoking

When asked "What makes you want to continue smoking?", the majority of respondents said it was craving (32.87%).

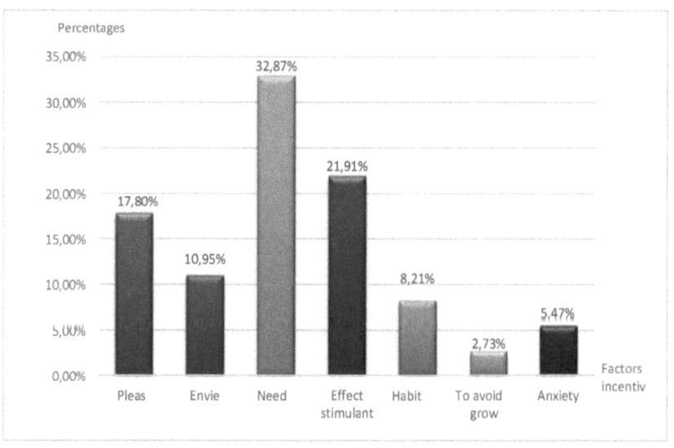

Figure 19: Factors that encourage people to continue smoking.

4.3. Quantity of tobacco

Daily smokers consume an average of 14 cigarettes a day (15 cigarettes a day for men and 8 cigarettes a day for women). The average pack/year (PA) of cigarettes consumed was 5 PA, with extremes ranging from 0.5 to 13 PA.

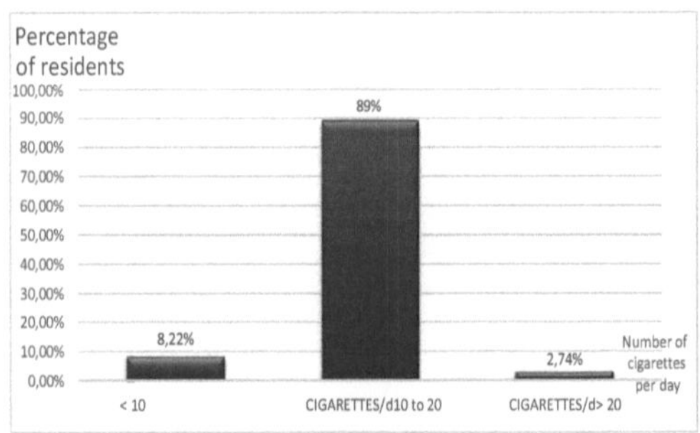

Figure 20: Amount of tobacco smoked per day.

4.4.Forms of tobacco used

Cigarettes were the form of tobacco most smoked by 71 residents. Only one resident used chicha or cigars. The type of consumption is specified in the following table:

Table VI: Types of tobacco consumed.

Shapes	Workforce	Percentage (%)	
Cigarette	73	100	
Cigar	1	1,4	
Chicha	1	1,4	
Total	73	100	

4.5. Associated substances

Smoking can be a factor in the initiation of other substances. For example, one resident admitted to using cannabis and 29 others to using alcohol.

Table VII: Substances associated with tobacco.

	Workforce	Percentages (%)
Alcohol	29	39,7
Cannabis	1	1,4
No	43	58,9
Total	73	100

4.6. Place of smoking

The majority of residents who smoked consumed their cigarettes in tea rooms and cafés (76.7%). However, 11 residents also smoke in hospital, which is equivalent to 15% of residents who smoke. No residents smoke in front of their patients.

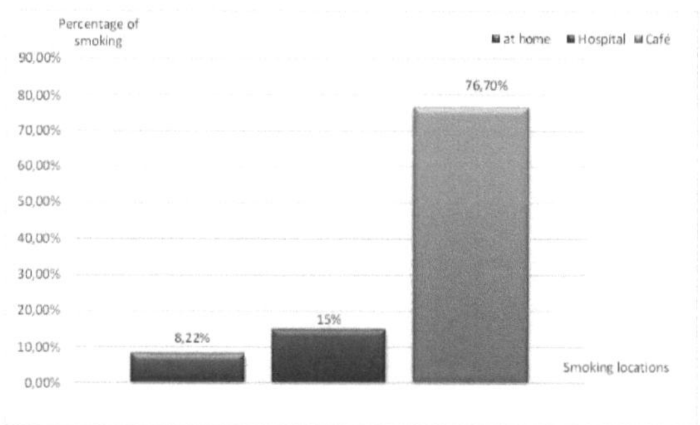

Figure 21: Main place of smoking.

4.7. Level of dependence

The Fagerstrom scale used to assess dependence produced the following results:

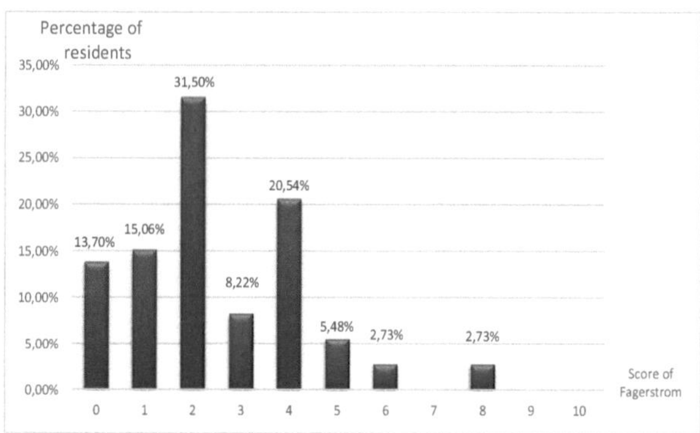

Figure 22: Residents' level of dependence on tobacco according to the Fagerstrom test score.

We noted that 65.8% of smokers said they smoked their first cigarette within 60 minutes of waking up and 1% between 6 and 30 minutes after waking up. The degree of dependence on tobacco is specified below:

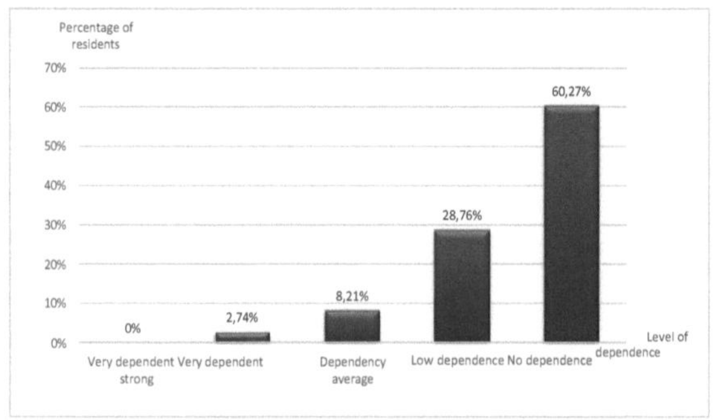

Figure 23: Breakdown of dependency levels.

5. Subsequent attitudes of residents who smoke

5.1. Towards their smoking habits

5.1.1 Wanting to stop smoking

Only 8.22% of resident smokers had a strong desire to stop smoking at the time of the survey.

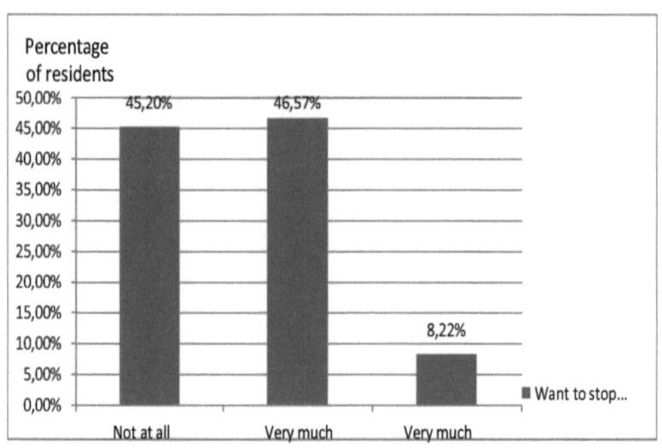

Figure 24: Current attitudes towards smoking among residents who smoke.

5.1.2 After 1 month

After 1 month, 67% of smokers think they will continue to smoke as much.

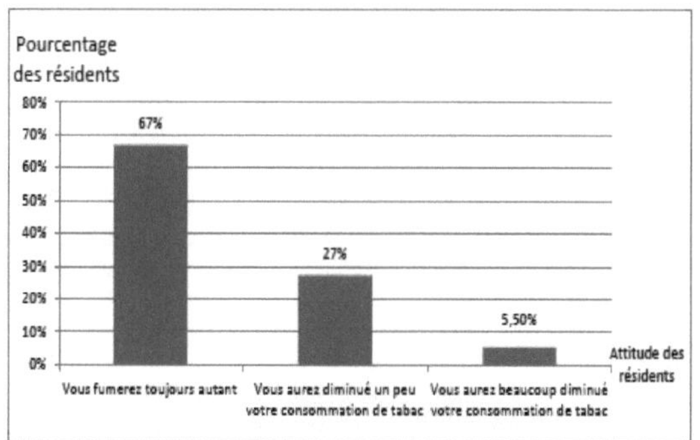

Figure 25: Smoking habits of residents after 1 month.

5.1.3 After 6 months

After 6 months, 54.8% of smokers think they will continue to smoke as much as before.

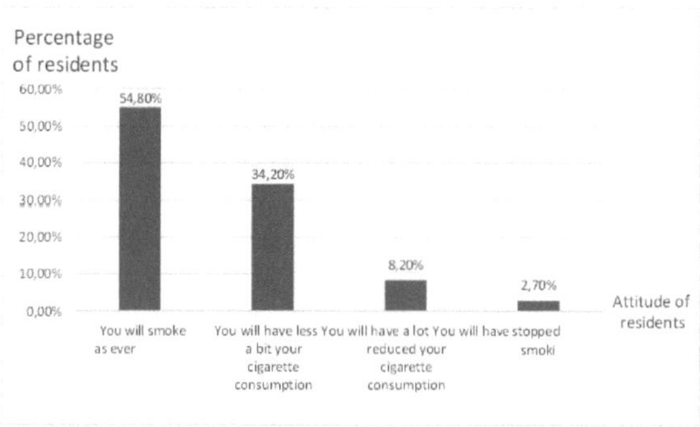

Figure 26: Smoking attitudes of residents after 6 months.

5.2. Towards their patients' smoking habits

5.2.1. Minimum advice practice

We noted that 158 residents were prepared to give their patients minimal advice as a matter of course, i.e. 71.70% of all residents surveyed. There was no statistically significant relationship between patient counselling and residents' smoking status.

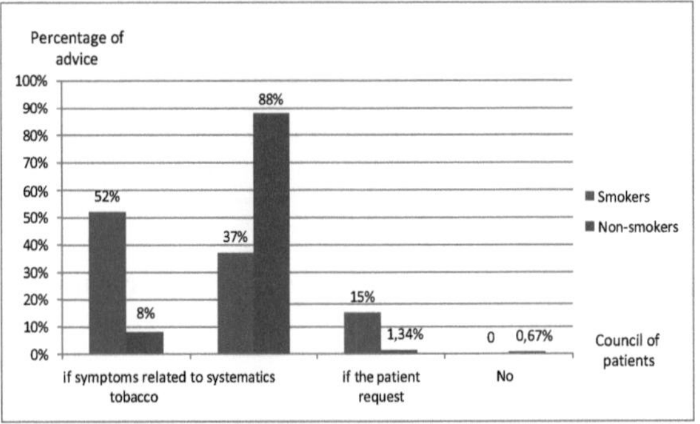

Figure 27: Patient advice on smoking.

5.2.2. Ability to convince smokers to stop smoking

We noted that 86.3% of smoking residents believe they have sufficient knowledge to convince patients who want to stop smoking.

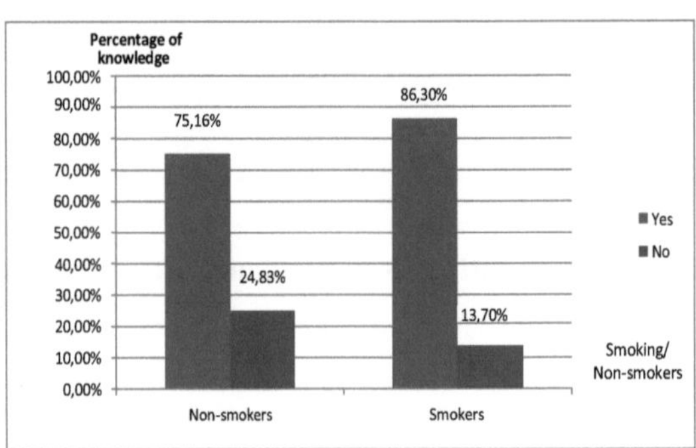

Figure 28: Residents' knowledge of how to convince their patients to stop smoking.

6. Weaning

6.1. Wishing to wean off

To the question "What do you think your chances are of giving up smoking?", using a numerical scale graduated from 0 to 100, the majority of residents marked the value 40, which means that the chances are less than half.

Table VIII: Smoking residents' percentage chances of quitting smoking.

Chances (%)	Workforce	Percentage (%)
10	9	12,3
20	7	9,6
30	12	16,4
40	17	23,3
50	11	15,1
60	7	9,6
70	4	5,5
80	2	2,7
90	2	2,7
100	2	2,7
Total	73	100

6.2. Withdrawal attempts

It was noted that 29 residents had tried weaning at least once. Only one resident tried 7 times with constant failure.

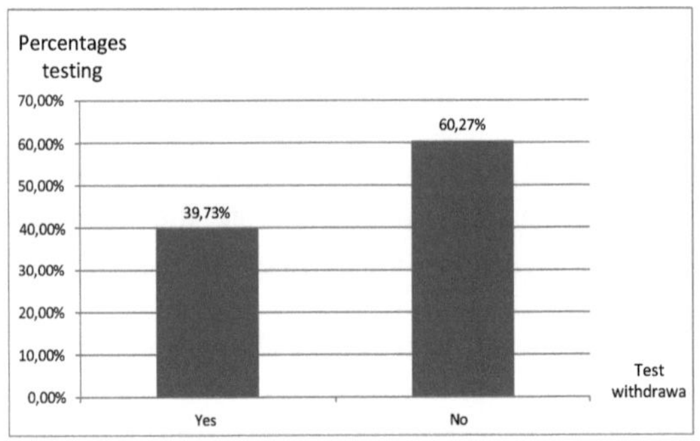

Figure 29: Stop smoking test.

6.3. Maximum duration of successful withdrawal attempts

The average duration of successful withdrawal attempts was 36 days, with extremes ranging from 1 day to 4 years. Three residents have managed to quit smoking and are now considered ex-smokers.

6.4. Weaning methods

When trying to give up smoking, the residents mainly used electronic cigarettes (3 cases). The majority of residents did not use any specific treatment

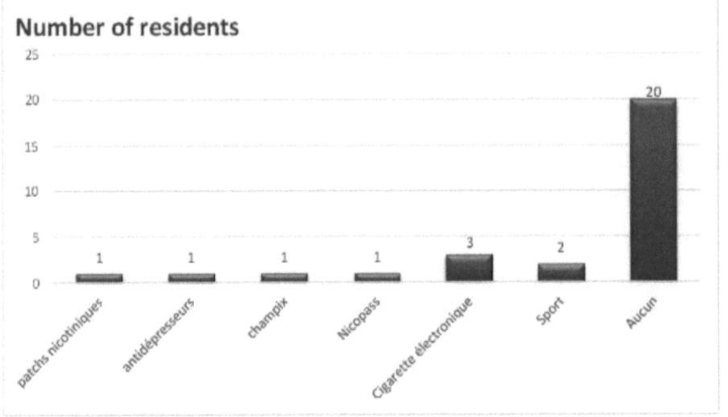

Figure 30: Smoking cessation methods.

6.5. Factors encouraging withdrawal

Of the 29 residents who wanted to stop smoking, 24 attributed this to their knowledge of tobacco-related illnesses. The price of a box of cigarettes to encourage people to give up smoking is between 10 and 32 dinars

Table IX: Factors encouraging smoking cessation.

	Workforce	Percentage (%)
Knowledge of tobacco-related diseases	24	88.90
Inconvenience to family and friends	1	3.70
Drug effect	2	7.40
Tobacco prices	2	7.40

7. Residents' knowledge of the pathologies caused by smoking. Smoking and non-smoking residents were given a series of pathologies to identify those that could be linked to smoking.

Table X: Residents' knowledge of diseases caused by smoking.

Smokers			Non-Smokers	
The role of tobacco	Determinant (%)	Non-determinant (%)	Determinant (%)	No determinant (%)
Bladder cancer	96.89	3.11	96.64	3.35
Diseases coronary	100	0	100	0
Cancer bronchial	100	0	99.3	0.7
COPD	98.63	1.37	100	0
Arteritis	95.89	4.11	97.3	2.7
Laryngeal cancer	94.52	5.48	92.61	7.4
Leukoplakia of the mouth and lips	48	52	61	39

8. Residents' views on certain aspects of tobacco control

8.1. Complete ban on tobacco advertising

The majority of both groups are in favour of banning tobacco advertising.

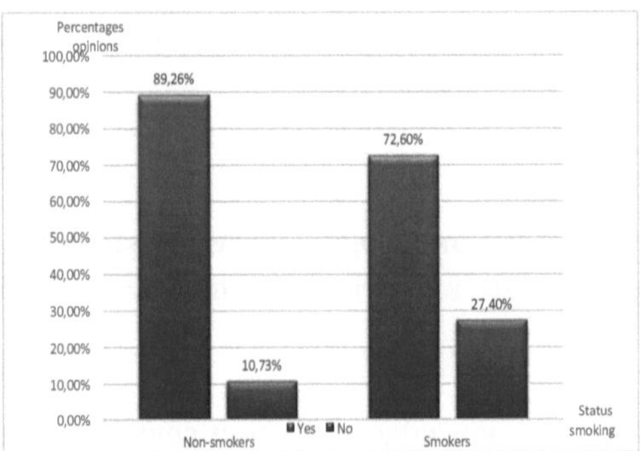

Figure 31: Residents' opinions on a complete ban on tobacco advertising.

8.2. Ban on smoking in public places

More than 95% of all residents in the 2 groups were in favour of banning smoking in public places, with no significant difference between the 2 groups.

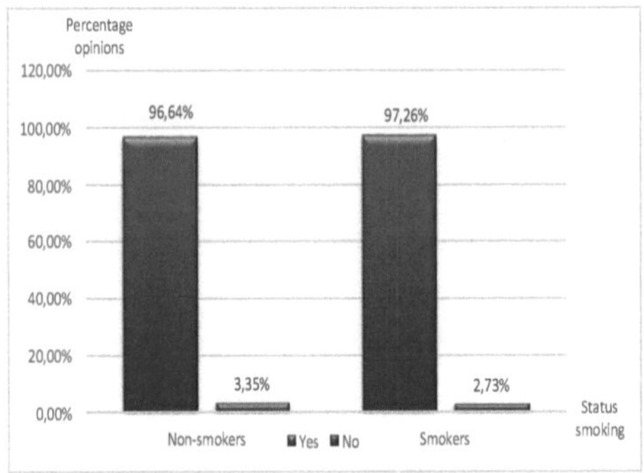

Figure 32: Residents' opinions on the ban on smoking in enclosed public places.

8.3. Ban on smoking in hospitals

The ban on smoking in hospitals was reported by almost all residents, regardless of their smoking status.

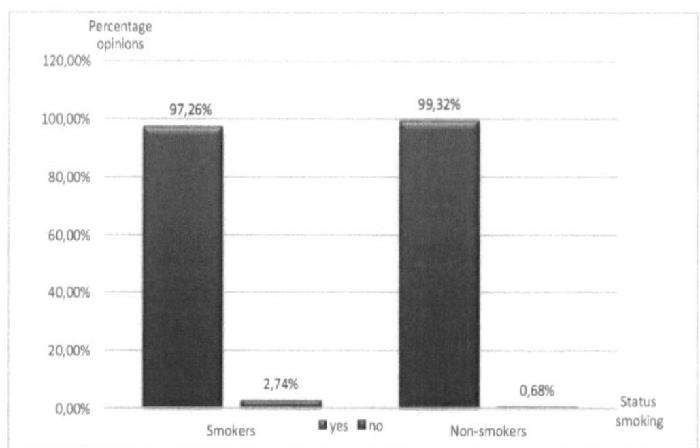

Figure 33: Residents' views on an absolute ban on smoking in hospitals.

8.4.Residents' views on training healthcare staff to help people give up smoking.

It was noted that all the residents were in favour of training healthcare staff to help them stop smoking.

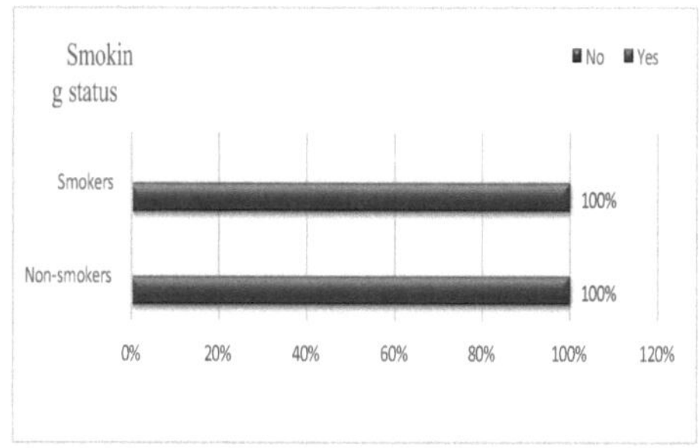

Figure 34: Residents' opinions on the training of medical and paramedical staff to help people stop smoking.

DISCUSSION

1. Analysis of participation

Overall participation in the study was good (78%). This testifies to the interest shown by residents in the subject of smoking. A study carried out in France among medical interns in the Poitou-Charentes region on smoking among interns showed that 406 medical interns out of a total of 649 responded to the questionnaire, giving an overall participation rate of 62.6 % **[9].** A variation was noted depending on the speciality, as shown in the following table:

Table XI: Comparison between our study and a French study concerning the percentage of participation in the study.

Specialities	Our study (%)	French study (%)
Intensive care anaesthesia	52.6	61
Medical biology	81.57	77
Obstetrics and gynaecology	93	65
Occupational medicine	100	100
Paediatrics	68	56
Psychiatry	89	65.9
Medical specialities	79	45.6
Surgical specialities	76	66.4
Total	77.89	62.6

2. Epidemiology

2.1.Prevalence of smoking

Over the past thirty years, studies have shown that the smoking epidemic is real in Tunisia and that prevalence is high, particularly among men. However, most of the studies published on this subject have focused on very specific groups **[10-11].**

2.1.1. In the general population

The prevalence of smoking in the general population in Tunisia is 15%, as reported in 2013 **[12].** Other studies have been published on consumption of tobacco in Tunisia concerning of populations populations,such as regional populations (a semi-urban community in the Tunisian Sahel **[13]** and the governorate of Greater Tunis - Ariana **[14].** In Maghreb countries such as Algeria and Morocco, prevalence rates were 26% and 28.6% respectively **[15-16].**

Table XII: Geographical distribution of smoking prevalence.

Population studied	Year of study	Prevalence (%)
General Tunisian population [12]	2013	15,2
City of Sousse [17]	2005	28
Algeria [15]	2009	26
Morocco [16]	2005	28,6

2.1.2. With doctors

Doctors usually play a vital role in changing the smoking behaviour of smokers **[18-19].** However, having doctors who smoke is bound to have a negative impact on the way patients view their doctors. The study of smoking among doctors began in the 1950s. In the UK, smoking among doctors has been studied in several longitudinal and prospective studies showing an increase in its frequency **[20-21].** In Tunisia, smoking by doctors has also been studied since 1980, mainly among general practitioners. At that time, prevalence was 53% among GPs **[22].**

2.1.3. For medical students

Smoking among medical students has been extensively evaluated by several national and international studies.In Tunisia, this scourge is on the increase. This table summarises all the studies relating to smoking by medical students.

Table XIII: Smoking among medical students.

References	Year of study	Prevalence (%)	Special features of the population
Fakhfakh R. et al [23]	1989	27,1	
	1997	33	
Fakhfakh R. et al [24]	1996	24,1	First year
		37,1	end of studies
			medical
M Ndiaye. et al [25]	2001	76,76	
Ghannem H. et al [26]	2004-2005	19.2	
Ben Salah N. et al [27]	2010	62,5	Men
		31,8	women
S. Alzayani, R.	2011	24.8	male
Hamadeh [28]		9.1	women
C. Zedini et al [29]	2012-2013	21.8	

2.1.4. For interns

Several studies have been carried out to assess the prevalence of smoking among residents, given the key role played by this group in patient management. Three studies are summarised in the table below.

Table XIV: Prevalence of smoking, studies of interns in France, Algeria and Tunisia.

References	Year study	Prevalence of smoking (%)
L. Salomon et al [30].	2000	36
O. Saighi et al [31].	2007	19.1
Yann Brabant [32].	2011	28.8

2.1.5. For residents

The profile of interns and residents is intermediate between medical students and specialist doctors. Few studies have assessed smoking among residents. Of those that have, a French study estimated the prevalence of smoking among residents at 45.7% in men and 25% in women **[33].** A second study showed that the prevalence of resident smokers at the Poitou-Charentes University Hospital was 28% **[32].** The prevalence observed in our study (32.88%) is much closer to that of specialist doctors than that of interns, which corresponds well to the actual situation of a resident in our country.

2.1.6. With senior citizens

The study of smoking among healthcare professionals showed that, among doctors, smoking behaviour was significantly influenced by grade. The most frequent smokers were associate lecturers, with a smoking prevalence of 39% **[34].**

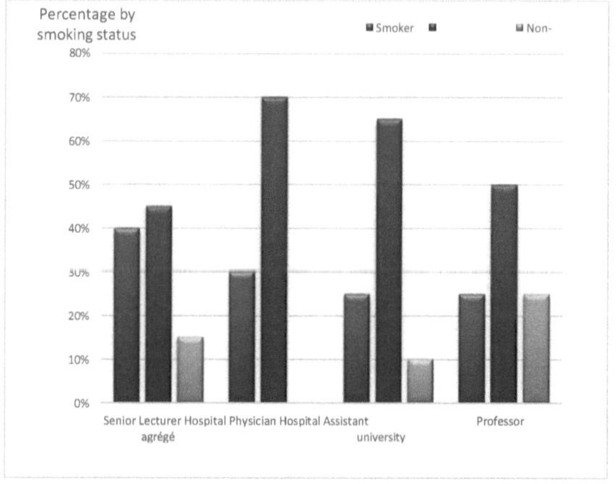

Figure 35: Smoking among senior citizens.

It is also lower than that observed in a population of comparable age, i.e. 7.1% in women and 54.8% in men (nurses and care assistants **[35].**
In our study, smoking among residents was estimated at 32.88%.

3. Characteristics of residents who smoke

3.1.Age of smoking initiation

In order to obtain information on residents' smoking history, it was preferable to interview residents since their initiation of smoking. The age of initiation was between 14 and 18 (63% of the population) **[35].** The average age of smoking initiation among residents was 22 years, with extremes ranging from 12 to 25 years.

3.2. Gender

Several Tunisian studies **[36-39]** report a male predominance. The relative rarity of smoking among women may be linked to the explicit or implicit socio-familial disapproval of such behaviour in women, and probably also to the association in the collective imagination between smoking and female promiscuity. For the same reasons, it could be assumed that such behaviour was under-reported by women.

4. Factors influencing residents' smoking habits

4.1 Stress

In our study, the most common reason for the first cigarette was stress (49.3%). Then came pleasure and the effect of friends and family in respectively 19.2% and 16.4% of cases. This is completely different for young people of the same age in different professions, and even for residents. These results testify to the importance of the psychological stress experienced by residents.

Table XV: Smoking initiation by population.

Incentive factors	Stress (%)	Pleasure (%)	Surroundings (%)	Concentration (%)	Keeping the weight off (%)	Anxiety (%)	Advertising (%)
External [40]	12	36	17	2	1	20	.
Internal [41]	14.7	18	8	.	2	10	28
Residents [42]	49.3	19.2	16.4	8.2	1.3	4.1	.

4.2 Family and friends smoking

Smoking by family and friends was identified as a risk factor for teenage smoking. The literature has clearly demonstrated the influence of parents, siblings and friends on the initiation of smoking in children **[43-44],** particularly through social learning mechanisms **[45].**

This was not the case for residents. In our study, the presence of smokers in the community had no statistically significant influence on smoking or non-smoking status. Paradoxically, the residents who had a larger number of smokers were non-smokers.

4.3 Influence of cigarette prices

Raising the price of cigarettes has long been seen as an effective way of reducing smoking among young people. This was not the case with residents, where this measure would have no effect on their consumption. This can be explained by the high degree of dependence which, whatever measure is taken, will have no effect on consumption. It can also be explained by the degree of financial autonomy that the residents have, since they have their own income.

4.4 Influence of medical studies

Medical studies had a major influence on the smoking status of smokers.

4.4.1 Influence of the externship period

We noted that 58 residents were influenced by the externship period in increasing their smoking, i.e. 79.45% of all residents who smoked. This testifies to the influence of medical studies as an initiating factor in stress and fatigue, so externals feel the need to smoke.

4.4.2 Influence of the internship period

The internship is an important stage in the professional life of any general practitioner or specialist. During this period, the doctor is directly confronted with patients and begins to acquire responsibilities. This transitional phase between theoretical medical studies and the practice of medicine is often awkward and stressful for most interns, especially at the beginning. A number of particular features of this period can be noted.

4.4.2.1 Mental health of interns

However, a number of studies carried out over the last ten years **[46-48],** some of which dealt with the burnout syndrome **[46], provide an overview of the** psychological health of interns and their lifestyle. The result was that this was a phase when interns were at risk of stress, fatigue and burn-out, most often linked to their training, confrontation with suffering and work overload.

4.4.2.2 Consumption of psychoactive substances

With regard to the lifestyles of interns, Jérémie Chirario studied the consumption of psychoactive substances by 527 Parisian medical interns (268 general medicine interns and 259 speciality interns) **[47].** Alcohol was found to be the most commonly used substance. Tobacco was the second most commonly used substance and 45% of them had increased their consumption during their internship. 41% of interns said they used nothing. Similarly, Julien Hérault's work, also devoted to the use of psychoactive substances, but among medical interns at the faculties of Lyon and Angers **[48]** found the same results. Concerning alcohol, 20% of interns said they had drunk alcohol. to relieve their stress.The intern will therefore look for anti-stress solutions, including taking up smoking or increasing cigarette consumption. This was confirmed in our study, since 83.5% of residents who smoked reported that their smoking had increased during the internship period. This encourages us to familiarise externs as much as possible with the practical side of medicine in order to avoid this additional stress at the beginning of the internship period.

4.4.2.3 Financial independence

Similarly, this is the first salary a doctor receives during his or her career. This means that interns are no longer dependent on their parents and therefore find it easier to buy cigarettes.

4.4.3 Influence of residency period

4.4.3.1 Influence of the residency competition

The residency examination is a national competition that allows successful candidates to specialise. The competition is so stressful that some describe it as "inhuman", to emphasise the degree of stress it causes candidates. This competition was responsible for an increase in smoking among 91.7% of residents. Only 8.3% succeeded in controlling their smoking when preparing for the residency competition. It would therefore be interesting to raise awareness among externs, particularly men, who may be more vulnerable, about controlling their smoking during this very anxiety-provoking period of their training.

4.4.3.2 Influence of level of education

In our study, the number of smokers was highest in the first 2 years of specialty training. This shows that residents start their specialty with an embarrassing level of stress, which they try to overcome by smoking. The further they progress in their specialty, the more they discover it and the less stress they experience.

4.4.3.3 Influence of speciality

Medical specialities vary, and many of them are more demanding, particularly those involving surgery or intensive care. Theoretically, these stressful specialties should include a much larger number of smokers than medical or basic specialties. This was true in our study, where the number of smokers was 73.33% in surgical specialties and only 16.66% in basic science specialties.

4.4 Influence of the number of hours worked per day

According to our study, contrary to what we thought, the residents who worked the most were non-smokers. This can be explained as follows:

- Either that, or that residents who work more have no time to waste in tea rooms and consequently smoke.
- Either smokers experience a drop in productivity, probably because of the harmful effects of tobacco.

4.5 Influence of the number of shifts per month

Doctors have often described on-call duty as a source of stress. This has led them to look for solutions to overcome this stress and stay awake. The simplest and best-known solution is smoking. This was noted in a French study in which several activities encouraged smokers to smoke more, including on-call duty in 90.3% of cases **[49].**

In our study, the percentage of smokers increased with the number of shifts per month, peaking at 7 and 8 shifts. Without shifts, the percentage of smokers was minimal (10.3%). Between 10 and 12 shifts, only 1% were smokers. This is explained by the small number of residents in this interval.

5. Characteristics of smoking

5.1 Forms of tobacco used

Tobacco comes in two forms: smoked tobacco and smokeless tobacco. The most commonly consumed form of smoked tobacco is cigarettes. This was also true in our population, where 97.3% of residents who smoked consumed cigarettes. A study of the behaviour, knowledge and attitudes of hospital staff at Mohamed V Hospital in Meknes with regard to smoking showed that the prevalence of consumption of other tobacco products breaks down as follows **[49]:** cigars are consumed by 11.5% of current smokers, the same rate for pipes (11.5%), followed by shisha (7.7%).Tobacco, whatever form it takes, contains numerous toxic substances and is highly addictive, leading to chronic use that is harmful to health **[50].**Cigarettes are still the most widely smoked tobacco product in the world, the most effective at delivering nicotine and the most toxic to health. Approximately ninety per cent of lung cancers in men are attributable to smoking, and cardiovascular diseases and respiratory diseases are the second and third leading causes of death among smokers respectively **[51].**

Roll-your-own tobacco, which is less expensive than manufactured cigarettes, is most often used by young men on low incomes who are highly addicted to tobacco. A study in the UK showed that tar and nicotine levels were higher in 57% and 77% of roll-your-own tobacco smokers respectively, compared with smokers of manufactured cigarettes **[52]. Rolling tobacco is** also commonly used to consume cannabis, the pulmonary toxicity of which is strongly suspected **[53].**

5.2 Smoking locations

The ban on smoking in public places has helped to reduce smoking among smokers. This is not always the case, however, as 15% of resident smokers also smoke in hospital, but never in front of their patients. Quite apart from the sympathy we may feel for this or that behaviour, it is vital, as those responsible for the day-to-day lives of the people entrusted to doctors, to tackle this problem of cohabitation. in a rational manner. "While smoking may sometimes be tolerated in certain places, the constant concern to ensure the protection of non-smokers is a priority" **[54].**

5.3 Associated substances

Smoking is a gateway to the use of other substances, particularly alcohol and cannabis. So it was not surprising to find 29 cases of alcoholism and one case of cannabis use in our population. This represents only reported cases. The reality is certainly different.

5.3.1 Alcohol addiction

There are many similarities between alcohol and tobacco addiction. Not all smokers are alcohol-dependent or only alcohol abusers, but smokers who consume alcohol generally drink more than non-smokers; not all alcohol consumers, whether abusers or not, necessarily become alcohol-dependent, but more than 80% of alcohol-dependent patients are smokers and heavily dependent on tobacco **[55-56].** Smoking cessation in alcohol-dependent patients remains difficult: the cessation of smoking in alcohol-dependent patients is generally not sustainable if the patient's alcohol dependence is not treated beforehand or at the same time (existence of reciprocal conditioning). These patients generally find it more difficult to stop smoking than drinking; on the other hand, stopping smoking in a weaned alcoholic does not encourage them to start drinking again. They require treatment in an alcoholology unit **[57], and** the identification of abusers and alcohol-dependents can benefit from the use of various tests: DATA, AUDIT **[55].**

5.3.2 Cannabis addiction

Drug use was reported by only one resident. This shows that cannabis use is rare in the socio-professional category of residents and doctors in general.

5.4 Level of dependence

When we assessed dependency using the Fagerstrom scale **(Appendix 2),** we found that 60% of residents were not dependent. This is interesting in terms of smoking cessation.

5.4.1 Definition of dependency

The WHO defines substance dependence as: "A state, psychic and sometimes physical, resulting from the interaction between a living organism and a substance, characterised by behavioural or other responses that always include a compulsion to take the substance regularly or periodically in order to feel its psychic effects and sometimes to avoid the discomfort of its absence (withdrawal) **[65].**

5.4.2 Fagerstrom test

Physical dependence can be assessed simply by means of a self-administered questionnaire: the Fagerström test. This is a simple six-question test with a total score ranging from zero to ten. Dependence is deemed to be strong if the score is equal to or greater than six.

5.4.3 Dependency factors

Addiction is the result of a combination of personal vulnerability (genetic and/or acquired), one or more substances with psychoactive effects, and a socio-cultural environment. Together, these factors create a complex interrelationship that combines biological sensations, emotions, cognition and the environment, and presides over the development of addiction. The latter involves the brain's reward system. The INSERM collective report (2004) set out the various elements of this addiction **[58].** Smoking is a behaviour **[59]** that is acquired and maintained, reinforced by numerous internal or environmental stimuli. In addition to a psycho-behavioural dependence, there is a pharmacological dependence in which nicotine plays a central role. This dependence is influenced by a number of factors, detailed below.

5.4.3.1 Pharmacological dependence

Like all addictive substances, it is responsible for psychostimulant functions and reinforcing effects, and induces self-administration behaviour in animals and craving in humans. Deprivation causes withdrawal symptoms that are corrected by administration of this substance **[60].** Inhalation of smoke results in a massive supply of nicotine ("bolus effect") which reaches the brain in a few seconds and saturates the receptors within a few minutes, causing both a temporary deactivation of these receptors and up-regulation (increase in the number of receptors or reduced turnover). The short half-life of nicotine (2 to 4 hours on average) encourages the onset and development of dependence **[61].**

Other substances present in tobacco smoke, such as β-carbolines (harmane, norharmane) or those synthesised endogenously, have an MAOI-like action (MAO activity in the brains of heavy smokers is reduced by 40 There is in fact a contrast between the weak reinforcing powers of nicotine in animals and the strong dependence on tobacco in humans **[62].** Nicotine, among other factors, interferes with the brain's reward system, made up of dopaminergic modulator neurons linking numerous structures: ventral tegmental area, prefrontal cortex, amygdala, nucleus accumbeus in which all addictive substances, including tobacco, cause an increase in dopamine levels. All the information processed by the reward system converges in the hypothalamus **[58].** As well as dopamine, other neurotransmitters seem to be involved, such as norepinephrine, serotonin, acetylcholine, gamma-aminobutyric acid, glutamic acid and endogenous opioids.

5.4.3.2 Genetic vulnerability factors

Genetic vulnerability factors interact with various environmental and behavioural factors. These genetic factors influence the activity of cytochrome P450 (CYP2A6), the main oxidising pathway (80%) for nicotine, which distinguishes between "slow and fast metabolisers", as well as the number and nature of nicotine receptors, and the nature and organisation of dopaminergic, noradrenergic and serotonergic receptors and pathways. These variations concern both the nature and organisation of nicotinic receptors in the dopaminergic, noradrenergic and serotonergic pathways. Genetic factors also influence psychological vulnerability, the appearance or development of psychopathologies, tobacco dependence and response to treatment to help people stop smoking **[58].**

5.4.3.3 Environmental factors

The subject's adaptation to his or her environment involves constant remodelling of neuronal networks, which may be altered by nicotine, explaining both the extent of dependence in some people and the difficulty of withdrawal **[58, 63 and 64], and** the fact that prenatal exposure to tobacco may induce vulnerability to smoking **[58].** There are many factors that facilitate or maintain consumption **[58-59]:** environmental, relational and psychological factors, local sensory stimuli associated with inhalation (heat, irritation of the airways, pleasure of inhaling, olfactory or gustatory perceptions induced by various additives or flavouring agents such as menthol).

5.5 Subsequent attitudes of residents who smoke

5.5.1 Towards their smoking habits

However, numerous studies **[66-69]** have reported that medical students at the end of their studies are poorly prepared for this role and that their attitudes towards smokers depend on their personal smoking behaviour. Regarding smoking cessation, only 8.20% of smoking residents had a strong desire to stop smoking when they answered the questionnaire. After 1 month, 67% of smokers thought they would continue to smoke just as much. After 6 months, 54.8% of smokers think they will continue to smoke as much as before.

5.5.2 Towards their patients' smoking habits

The majority of residents, regardless of their smoking status, agreed to provide minimal advice to their patients who smoke. This shows that most of them are aware of the harmful effects of smoking and are ready to start the process of weaning their patients off tobacco.Only 1.35% of our residents adopt a passive attitude towards their future patient when the latter does not have a smoking-related illness. They are also less likely to intervene when they themselves are smokers. This passive attitude raises the question of the role of doctors as players in promoting health and preventing the risks of smoking. In other words, health promotion and education are not part of the students' conception of their medical field of practice, probably because of the inadequacy of medical training. It seems that medical studies have a definite impact on knowledge, but have no effect on behaviour.

6. Diseases caused by smoking

It has been clearly demonstrated that tobacco remains the main cause of bronchial cancer, with a dose-effect relationship **[70-73].** The role of smoking has been known for over 60 years. The quantity of tobacco smoked and the duration of smoking are the main factors, and the concept of "pack-years" takes these two parameters into account, even if the duration has a much greater impact than the quantity smoked per day. Smoking is a major cardiovascular risk factor. More than one in ten cardiovascular deaths worldwide can be attributed to smoking, making it the most important cause of avoidable cardiovascular mortality **[74].** It is the main and often isolated factor in acute coronary events in young people. More than 80% of people presenting with a myocardial infarction before the age of 45 are smokers **[75].** There is no threshold for smoking intensity or duration, even for moderate or low levels of smoking **[76],** or for passive smoking **[77].** Its suppression can very quickly provide effective and significant protection **[78-79].** The INTERHEART study recently confirmed that, universally, smoking is the second most important risk factor for myocardial infarction, just behind dyslipidemia **[80].** All the essential data that every doctor needs to know about the coronary effects of smoking are contained in an analysis of this study specifically devoted to the results concerning tobacco **[81].**

There is a link between smoking and oral health. Tobacco consumption is the main risk factor for oral cancer **[82].** There is a causal relationship between smoking and cancers of the larynx, oesophagus, pharynx and cancers of the oral cavity such as cancer of the lip, cheek and gum **[83,84].**

Epidemiological studies show that smoking increases the risk of developing oral cancer by 5 to 9 times **[85].** Chewing tobacco and snuff are associated with a 50% increased risk of cancer of the gums, cheeks and inner lips, compared with the risk incurred by non-smokers **[82,83].** The risk of developing cancer of the cheek or gum is fifty times greater for long-term users of snuff **[83].** Consumption of smokeless products can lead to gingival recession, periodontal (gum) disease **[86]** and oral leukoplakia (white patches or lesions of the oral mucosa). Leukoplakia can transform dysplasia into cancer **[83].** An analysis of 18 publications favouring meta-analyses, large cohort studies and systematic reviews **[87-104]** indicates that active smoking increases hospital mortality by around 20% and major postoperative complications by 40% (deep infection, pneumonia, unscheduled intubation, pulmonary embolism, ventilation>48h, stroke, coma>24h, cardiac arrest, myocardial infarction, transfusion>5U, sepsis, septic shock).

7. Weaning

According to our study, more than half the residents have little chance of quitting smoking. This contradicts the low dependency rate already calculated by the Fagerstrom score.

7.1 Ability to convince smokers to stop smoking

The majority of residents in our study felt able to convince patients to stop smoking. This shows that smoking status has no influence on smoking cessation. Although the harmful effects of smoking are fairly well known, their knowledge of them is apparently not enough to dissuade children and teenagers from taking up smoking. The consequences of smoking seem very remote to young people. Many smokers want to stop, each for their own reasons, but they often fear that they won't succeed. Doctors can help their patients who smoke to express these reasons and support their motivation to change. The consultation is a good opportunity for smokers to express their wishes and expectations about quitting smoking, and to become aware of the risks involved. what they are going to have to give up. Residents can help them to identify their fears and ambivalence about smoking, so that they can be better supported.

7.2 Attempted withdrawal

According to our study, the number of withdrawal attempts is very similar to that of the general population of the same age. In Tunisia, 914 smokers took part in a descriptive cross-sectional study, targeting smokers who had taken part in awareness-raising days held in public places in Monastir and university establishments in the city of Monastir (engineering preparatory school, national engineering school, faculty of science, faculty of pharmacy and faculty of dentistry) **[105].** This study showed that more than 2/3 of them (70%) had made at least one quit attempt, the longest of which had lasted more than 6 months for 81 subjects (9%), and the last attempt had been made more than 6 months previously for 486 smokers (53%). These previous attempts were unaccompanied in 97% of cases. 2/3 of the smokers (67%) had a very strong desire to stop smoking, and 41% had very strong self-confidence in succeeding in their attempts. This study concluded that strong physical dependence is a main factor linked to the failure of attempts to quit smoking, the loss of self-confidence on the part of smokers to succeed in new attempts and, as a result, the maintenance of a fairly high prevalence of smoking in a country like Tunisia.

7.3 Duration of withdrawal attempts

According to a Tunisian study, the number of quit attempts and their duration were lower among Tunisian smokers than those described by Hyland in 2006 in the USA, Canada, England and Australia. This table summarises the number and duration of withdrawal attempts by country.

Table XVI: Number of withdrawal attempts by country.

	Never (%)	<= 1 week (%)	1 week and 6 months (%)	6 months or more (%)
Study Tunisian[105]	30	18	43	9
Canada [106]	27	39	47	52
UK [106]	20	30	34	38
Australia[106]	23	29	38	38
Thailand[107]	60	19	15	7
Malaysia[107]	47	44	5	4
France[108]	24	27	30	19
USA[106]	17	33	40	46

7.4 Factors encouraging withdrawal

Preventing a smoking-related health problem was the main reason for a previous attempt **[109-111].** Other factors encouraging cessation have been described in the literature, such as the presence of a young child in the family **[112],** pregnancy **[113]** and the presence of functional signs experienced by the subject and linked to smoking, confirming the value of minimal advice from any doctor **[111].** Other studies have shown that campaigns to raise awareness of the harmful effects of smoking encourage smokers to think about changing their smoking behaviour **[114]**, especially if these campaigns target disability and quality of life **[115].**

7.5 Factors in withdrawal failure

Smoking urges were the most feared adverse effects of withdrawal, and Filder had shown that they contributed to the failure of attempts to stop smoking **[116].** Heffner J **[117]** showed that they were at the root of continued consumption. A Tunisian study showed that the fear of excess weight following an improvement in appetite was reported by 27% of the subjects taking part in this study **[118]**. This fear was not influenced by the degree of dependence. In a prospective study conducted between 2004 and 2010, Kasteridis showed that weight gain was insignificant compared with the health benefits associated with smoking cessation, even in the obese population **[119].** In smokers, sleep disorders increased cardiovascular and cerebrovascular morbidity. In the course of smoking cessation, their management makes withdrawal less difficult and reduces the risk of relapse **[120].** A minority of smokers had sought medical help during previous attempts, and these smokers showed a high level of dependence and more signs of craving. These factors confirmed the need for treatment in subjects with a very high level of dependence. In this context, Vanasse proposed that healthcare professionals should consider tobacco as an addiction and take a specific approach to help based on age, gender and tobacco consumption **[121].** Torchalla insisted that treatments to help people stop smoking should be accessible even outside healthcare services **[122],** which will help to facilitate access to cessation methods, eliminate barriers between patients who smoke and cessation methods, and thus make action against smoking more effective.

8. The role of doctors in the patient withdrawal process

8.1 The role of nursing staff in the withdrawal process

All medical and paramedical staff in the hospital must be able to help smokers to stop smoking and must be involved in this support process. All patients should be systematically questioned about their smoking habits and their smoking status should be regularly recorded in their medical records. To achieve this, all nursing staff need to be trained in "advice on how to stop smoking". Healthcare staff also need to know how to prescribe nicotine substitutes quickly and organise effective care on each ward.

8.2 Proposed resources

To make it easier to identify and deal with smokers in each department or unit, we can :

- Strengthen tobacco education during medical studies and continuing medical education to improve the management of patients who smoke **[123].**
- Make every effort to separate the help that doctors should give their patients who smoke from their personal smoking habits.
- Train all healthcare staff to provide advice on quitting smoking and prescribing nicotine substitutes.
- Make a single "First Day Procedure" type form available in each care unit, so that nicotine substitutes can be identified and prescribed quickly.
- Make nicotine replacement therapies permanently available in sufficient quantities in every department.

8.3 Medical training

Continuing education is an obligation for hospital staff and healthcare professionals.Lifelong professional training is an obligation for all hospital staff. All healthcare professionals must provide evidence of their commitment to a continuous professional development programme involving continuous training, analysis, evaluation and improvement of their practices and management. risks. A commitment to an accreditation process is equivalent to a commitment to continuous professional development. The fight against smoking is a priority for healthcare professionals and continuing education.Training is an essential tool for the smoking cessation strategy The smoking cessation strategy must include staff training. Training in smoking cessation and smoking cessation advice is a key factor in ensuring that staff adopt a proactive attitude, provide the necessary advice and ensure effective smoking prevention. Without training, staff are tempted to respond only to questions asked by the patient who smokes, rather than initiating the discussion themselves. It is therefore essential for the hospital to have professionals who are aware of the problem of smoking. This training can be based on continuing education, in-house training and self-training. As part of continuing professional development, healthcare staff could be invited to choose training courses on tobacco and cessation assistance.Staff could also be offered the opportunity to take a university diploma in tobacco studies.To train a large number of staff over a short period of time, in-house training courses should be considered, which could be included in the school's training plan to validate their institutional nature and facilitate their implementation. These courses will focus on how to deal with smokers in hospital and in everyday life, and will cover identification, brief intervention, simplified procedures for treatment and referral, risk reduction, etc. It is important that all the training courses offered should be updated, for example every 5 years, so that they include new medical developments and are up to date.

8.4 The role of tobacco specialists

Where appropriate, we will be able to call on the establishment's tobaccologists/addictologists and thus have the possibility of training, assisting and advising carers in the health establishment's various non-addictive care departments or structures on issues of screening, diagnosis, management and referral of patients with addictive behaviour".

8.5 Training for medical interns and residents

Intervening with students in training and in training institutes is currently a necessity. The establishment will ensure that medical interns are trained in how to deal with smokers, which could be done at meetings at the start of their internship and residency.

CONCLUSION

Smoking is currently a major public health problem in Tunisia and throughout the world, responsible for a fairly high morbidity and mortality rate. According to the World Health Organisation (WHO), the death rate attributable to smoking is 5.4 million smokers a year. This rate is rising steadily, particularly in developing countries. In fact, the WHO report on the global tobacco epidemic in 2017 showed that 11.4% of young Tunisians aged between 13 and 15 and 24.9% of Tunisian adults are smokers. This scourge is currently affecting younger and younger people. Efforts should therefore be made at all levels to control the smoking epidemic in our country.In the fight against smoking, it has been well established that in order to reduce smoking, healthcare professionals (HCPs) must be at the forefront and that their role is critical. The code of practice adopted by the WHO in 2004 encourages HCPs to set an example by not smoking and to play an active part in the fight against smoking. As a result, all healthcare professionals are concerned and have a duty to warn their patients of the many risks they run by smoking. They must do their utmost to help patients give up smoking. They must be the first to set a good example, to refrain from smoking and to play an active part in the fight against smoking. In this context, minimum advice on quitting smoking is an essential part of smoking prevention. Minimal advice on quitting smoking is a brief, systematic intervention that any doctor can provide when in the presence of a smoker during a consultation. Advising patients to stop smoking is an important task for all hospital staff. It is difficult to create an environment conducive to a healthy lifestyle without involving hospital staff and helping the smokers among them to quit their habit. All healthcare professionals have a role to play in this area, and they must be to avoid a lack of effectiveness and discredit among smokers. Medical residents are key contacts for patients and therefore have an essential role to play in preventing smoking. They have a key role to play in reducing smoking and its harmful effects. Residents must therefore make the fight against smoking an integral part of their activities. In this context, the aim of our study of residents at Sfax university hospitals was to determine the prevalence of smoking in this professional category, to assess their behaviour and attitudes towards smoking and to determine their role in the fight against tobacco. This was a cross-sectional study conducted over a 2-month period from 1 February 2016 to 31 March 2016. The study population consisted of residents of the Hedi Chaker and Habib Bourguiba university hospital centres (CHU) in Sfax, whatever their specialty: medical, surgical or basic sciences and practising during the first six months of 2016. Residents who partially completed the questionnaire were subsequently excluded from the study.The study subjects were divided into three groups. Group I included all smokers who smoked a tobacco product at least once a day. Group II included ex-smokers, i.e. those who had smoked in the past and had not smoked for more than a year. Group III was made up of non-smokers, i.e. those who had never smoked. These last two groups were subsequently merged.The study was carried out in the form of a questionnaire written in French and comprising two types of question: closed questions where the choice of answer is imposed from a list of proposals, and open questions where the practitioner is free to propose an answer. Four parts were identified in The questionnaire consisted of a common section dealing with the resident's identity, a section for smokers, a section for ex-smokers and a section for non-smokers. Residents were contacted in three stages: The first stage was devoted to providing information about the survey on a topical medical issue. The second stage involved residents who had agreed to take part. The third stage consisted of collecting the various completed copies after two days. Copies that had not been completed were not considered invalid. A second request to complete the questionnaire was made. The fourth stage consisted of recovering all the copies after 4 days of the first recovery. Copies not completed by this second time were considered invalid and thus excluded from the survey. The total number of residents in the Sfax university hospitals during the study period was 285. Of these, 277 agreed to take part in the survey. Of these, 222 answered the questionnaire correctly, giving an overall participation rate of 78%. This shows that residents are interested in the subject of smoking. Residents who did not reply to the questionnaire were divided into two categories: those who declined to take part in the study when first approached, of whom there were eight. There were 8 of them, and the reasons given were :

- Too many requests and not enough time to answer a questionnaire considered long (5 residents).
- Lack of interest in surveys (1 resident)
- No reason (2 residents)

The second category was represented by those who initially agreed to respond but who were not present on the day the questionnaires were distributed (48 residents) and those who responded but whose forms were incomplete and therefore unusable (7 residents). The average age of the residents included in the study was 28.38 years, with extremes ranging from 25 to 34 years. The two most common age groups were [27-28] and [28-29]. The highest percentage of residents surveyed were women (52.70%). Half of the residents were married at the time of the survey (52.7%). Married residents were distributed as follows: 20 smokers, 1 ex-smoker, 96 non-smokers.The majority of residents surveyed lived in Sfax (92.8%). The residents' year of study varied between 1st year and 5th year. The majority were in their 2nd year. The participating residents had medical specialities (123 residents), surgical specialities (60 residents) and basic specialities (36 residents).The residents included in our study were classified as "non-smokers" and "non-smokers". "The group of ex-smokers was included in the non-smokers group on the basis of the criteria set out in the methodology. The group of ex-smokers was included in the group of non-smokers because they had been smoking for 02 years or more. The prevalence of smoking among residents was 32.88%. The group of smokers was represented by 73 residents, 97.26% of whom were male. Several Tunisian studies have reported a male predominance.The relative scarcity of smoking among women may be linked to the explicit or implicit social and family disapproval of such behaviour, and probably also to the association in the collective imagination between smoking and female promiscuity. For the same reasons, it could be assumed that such behaviour was under-reported by women. The age group most affected was between 27 and 29. It was noted that 51% of single people were smokers and only 17% of married people were smokers.The majority of residents who smoked were in surgical specialties, with a prevalence of 73.33%. Medical specialties vary, and many of them are more restrictive, particularly those involving surgery or intensive care. Theoretically, these stressful specialties should include a much larger number of smokers than medical or basic specialties. This was true in our study, where the number of smokers was 73.33% in surgical specialties and only 16.66% in basic science specialties. The number of smokers was lowest among residents at the end of their speciality (4th and 5th years).The number of smokers was highest in the first two years of the specialty. This shows that residents start their specialty with an embarrassing amount of stress, which they try to overcome by smoking. The further they progress in their specialty, the more they discover it and the more their stress diminishes. Outside on-call duty, smokers worked less than non-smokers, with a statistically insignificant difference: $p = 0.87$.The majority of residents worked on-call. The average number of shifts per month for smokers was lower than for non-smokers, with a statistically significant difference: $p = 0$. The average age of smoking initiation was 22 years, with extremes ranging from 12 to 25 years. Several factors were assessed to determine their influence on smoking initiation, including stress and pleasure.The circle of residents who smoked included smokers who varied between father, mother, brother and partner. All the residents surveyed had smokers in their entourage (regardless of smoking status or sex), with no statistically significant difference). The literature has clearly demonstrated the influence of parents, siblings and friends on the initiation of smoking in children, particularly through social learning mechanisms. This was not the case for residents. In our study, the presence of family smokers had no statistically significant influence on smoking or non-smoking status. Fifty-eight residents were influenced by the clerkship period. The clerkship exam period increased smoking by 79.45% of all smoking residents. This indicates the influence of medical studies as an initiating factor in stress and fatigue, and thus the need for smoking.The majority of residents reported an increase in smoking at the time of their internship. Only 1.44% reported a decrease in their smoking during this period. This phase is at risk of stress, fatigue and burn-out for residents, most often linked to their training, confrontation with suffering and work overload.Passing the residency competition had a statistically significant influence on residents' smoking habits. This competition is so stressful that some describe it as "inhuman", to emphasise the degree of stress it generates in candidates. To the question "Has your tobacco consumption been influenced by the increase in the price of tobacco?", 97.3% of residents answered "no".The average age at which regular smoking began was 22, with extremes ranging from 14 to 25. When asked "What makes you want to continue smoking?", the majority of respondents said it was craving (32.87%).Daily smokers consumed an average of 14 cigarettes a day (15 cigarettes a day for men and 8 cigarettes a day for women).The average number of cigarettes consumed per pack per year (PA) was 5 PA, with extremes ranging from 0.5 to 13 PA. Cigarettes were the form of tobacco most smoked by 71 residents. Only one resident used chicha or cigars.Smoking can be a factor in the initiation of other substances. Smoking is a gateway to the use of other substances, particularly alcohol and cannabis. So it was not surprising to find 29 cases of alcoholism and one case of cannabis use in our population. This represents only reported cases. The reality is certainly different.The majority of residents who smoked consumed their cigarettes in tea rooms and cafés (76.7%). However, 11 residents also smoke in hospital, which is equivalent to 15% of residents who smoke. No residents smoke in front of their patients. The Fagerstrom scale used to assess dependence yielded the following results: 65.8% of smokers said they smoked their first cigarette after 60 minutes of waking up and 1% between 6 and 30 minutes after waking up. Only 8.22% of smoking residents had a strong desire to stop smoking at the time of the survey.After 1 month, 67% of smokers thought they would continue to smoke as much. After 6 months, 54.8% of smokers thought they would continue to smoke as much. We noted that 158 residents were prepared to give their patients minimal advice systematically, i.e. 71.70% of all residents surveyed. There is no statistically significant relationship between patient counselling and residents' smoking status. The consultation is a good opportunity for smokers to express their wishes and expectations regarding quitting smoking, and to become aware of what they will have to give up. The residents can help them to identify their fears and ambivalence about smoking, so that they can be better supported. We noted that 86.3% of smoking residents believe they have sufficient knowledge to convince patients who want to stop smoking.To the question "What do you think your chances are of giving up smoking?", using a numerical scale graduated from 0 to 100, the majority of residents put a mark on the value 40, which means that the chances are less than half. It was noted that 29 residents had tried to quit at least once. Only one resident had tried 7 times with constant failure. The average duration of successful withdrawal attempts was 36 days, with extremes ranging from 1 day to 4 years. Three residents succeeded in giving up smoking and were therefore considered to be ex-smokers.When trying to give up smoking, the residents used electronic cigarettes in only 3 cases. The majority did not use any specific treatment. Of the 29 residents who wanted to stop smoking, 24 said it was because they knew about tobacco-related illnesses.The price of a box of cigarettes to encourage smoking cessation ranged from 10 to 32 dinars. A series of pathologies was proposed to residents, smokers and non-smokers, in order to determine those that could be linked to smoking. The majority of both groups were in favour of banning tobacco advertising. More than 95% of all residents in both groups were in favour of banning smoking in public places, with no significant difference between the 2 groups. The ban on smoking in hospitals was reported by almost all residents, regardless of their smoking status. It was noted that all the residents were in favour of training healthcare staff to help them stop smoking. This shows that the majority of them are aware of the harmful effects of smoking and are ready to start the process of weaning their patients off tobacco.

BIBLIOGRAPHY

1. Official WHO website: http://www.who.int/fr/news-room/fact-sheets/detail/tobacco.

2. Jean-Charles Deybach, Delia Cozzolino. Free distribution of nicotine substitutes and smoking cessation. A 3-year observation at the Louis Mourier Hospital. 2008.

3. Mohamed Hsairi, Ahlem Gzara. Global Youth Tobacco Survey. 2010; National, ages 13-15.

4. National Survey of Morbidity and Access to Care (TAHINA). 2005- 06 ; National, ages 35-70.

5. Harrabi I, Ghannem H, Ben Abdeaziz A et al. Smoking in schools in Sousse. Tunisie. Rev Mal Respir 2002; 19 :311-4.

6. Hyland A, Borland R, Li Q, Yong HH, McNeill A, Fong GT, et al. Individual level predictors of cessation behaviours among participants in the International Tobacco Control (ITC) Four Country Survey. Tob Control. 2006; 15:83-94.

7. Sienkiewicz-Jarosz H, Zatorski P, Baranowska A, Ryglewicz D, Bienkowski P. Predictors of smoking abstinence after first-ever ischemic stroke: a 3-month follow-up. Stroke. 2009;40 :2592-3.

8. Schiller JS, Ni H. Cigarette smoking and smoking cessation among persons with chronic obstructive pulmonary disease. Am J Health Promot. 2006;20:319-23.

9. BRABANT MY. Medical interns and smoking. :80.

10. Ben Khelifa F. Morphological and biochemical characteristics and epidemiology of diabetes in the population of Tunis. Tunis Imprimerie officielle de la République tunisienne; 1979.

11. Ben Romdhane H. Les cardiopathies ischémiques, l'épidémie et ses déterminants, Vol. 1. Les facteurs de risque: Résultats d'une étude épidémiologique auprès de 5771 adultes tunisiens. Tunis: Institut national de Santé publique; 2001.

12. Doll R, Hill AB. The mortality of doctors in relation to their smoking habits. Br Med J, 1954, 1, 1451-1455.

13. Ghannem H, Limam K, Ben Abdelaziz A, Hadj Fredj A, Marzouki M. Risk factors for cardiovascular disease in a semi-urban community in the Tunisian Sahel. Revue d'épidémiologie et de santé publique 1992;40:108-12.

14. Ben Romdhane H. Les cardiopathies ischémiques, l'épidémie et ses

déterminants, vol. 1. Les facteurs de risque: résultats d'une étude épidémiologique auprès de 5771 adultes tunisiens. Tunis: Institut National de Santé Publique; 2001.
15. Fahima Hassine, Asma Sriha, Afifa Kobaa. Knowledge, attitudes and practices of Sayada high school students with regard to smoking.
La tunisie Medicale - 2016 ; Vol 94 (n°01) : 54-59

16. S. Cherquaoui, MA. Tazi, N. Chaouki. Report on the epidemiological survey of smoking among schoolchildren in Morocco. 2001.
17. Harrabi I, Ghannem H, Ben Abdeaziz A et al. Smoking in schools in Sousse. Tunisie. Rev Mal Respir 2002; 19 :311-4.
18. Rosen C, Ashley MJ. Smoking and the health profession: recognition and performance of roles. Can J Pub/ Health, 1978, 69, 399-06.
19. Adriaanse H, Van Reek J. Physicians' smoking and its exemplary effect. Scand J Prim Health Care, 1989, 7,193-196.
20. Doll R, Hill AB. The mortality of doctors in relation to their smoking habits. Br Med J, 1954, 1, 1451-1455.
21. Doll R, Peto R. Mortality in relation to smoking:20 years observations on male British doctors. Br Med J,1976, 2, 1525-1536.
22. Largue G, Branelle A, Lebargy F. La toxicologie du tabac. Rev Prat 1993;43:1203-7.
23. M-S Soltani, A. Bchir, Fakhfakh R. Medical students: smoking and health: a national survey.
24. Fakhfakh R et al. Cahiers Santé 1996; 6: 37-42. Smoking among medical students in Tunisia: trends in behaviour and attitudes.
25. Ndiaye M, Ndir M, Quantin X, Demoly P, Godard P, Bousquet J. Smoking habits, attitudes and knowledge of medical students at the Faculty of Medicine, Pharmacy and Odontostomatology in Dakar, Senegal. Rev Mal Respir. 2003;9.
26. Harrabi I, Ghannem H, Kacem M, Gaha R, Ben Abdelaziz A, Tessier JF. Medical students and tobacco in 2004: A survey in Sousse, Tunisia. Int J Tuberc Lung Dis. 2006;10:328-32.
27. Ben Salah Nabil et al. Survey on smoking in schools and universities in Tunisia. 2010;70.
28. S. Alzayani, R. Hamadeh. Tobacco Smoking among Medical Students in the Middle East. International Journal for Innovation Education and Research, 3(2).
29. C. Zedini, A. Ben Cheikh, M. Mallouli, M. Limam, J. Sahli, M. El Ghardallou, A. Mtiraoui, T. Ajmi. Prevalence and factors associated with

smoking among students in the city of Sousse (Tunisia). Eastern Mediterranean Health Journal; Jan2016, Vol. 22 Issue 1, p39-46, 8p.
30. Salomon L, LeVu S, Steffen C, Papy E, Blanchon T, Mathern G, Dautzenberg B, Delormas P, Brücker G. Residents and smoking: knowledge and practice.
31. O. Saighi, S. Abderrahim, N. Hadjer, L. Nacef, S.A. Lehachi. Smoking in the university medical environment. Study of 282 interns at the Faculty of Medicine of Blida O. Pneumology, CHU Blida, Blida, Algeria.
32. BRABANT MY. Medical interns and smoking. :80.
33. Mahmoudi A. Nancy medical school residents and smoking. 2003 ;108.
34. Khanchel F. Tabagisme des professionnels de la sante (etude sur 2000 professionnels de l'hopital charles nicolle). Thesis Med Tunis 2010.
35. Fakhfakh R, Hsairi M, Belaaj R, Romdhane H, Achour N. Epidemiology and prevention of smoking in Tunisia: current situation and outlook. 2001 ;9.
36. Becha F. Tabagisme et dépendance physique à la nicotine à l'adolescence. A study of 906 secondary school students in the Sidi Makhlouf district. Dissertation for the adolescentology master's degree. Sfax Faculty of Medicine. 2007/2008
37. Harrabi I, Ghannem H. Le tabagisme en milieu scolaire à sousse, tunisie. Rev mal Respir 2002; 19, 311-314.
38. Soltani Ms, Bchir A. Comportement tabagique et attitudes des étudiants en Médecine à monastir en regard du tabac (sahel tunisien). Rev mal respir 2000 ;17 : 77-82.
39. Rakam A. Factors associated with smoking among adolescents. A survey of 100 medical students. Dissertation for the Adolescentology Master's degree. Sfax Faculty of Medicine. 2007/2008
40. Smaoui Ben Abdelaziz S. Depression, Alexithymia And Smoking In Tunisian Students. Etude Cas/Temoin. Thesis Med Sfax 2015.
41. Brabant MY. Les Internes En Médecine Et Le Tabac. :80.

42. Mahmoudi A. Les Residents De La Faculte De Medecine De Nancy Et Le Tabac. 2003;108.
43. Devries H, Engels R, Kremers S, et al. Parents' and friends' smoking status as predictors of smoking onset: findings from six European countries. Health educ res 2003;18(5):627-636.
44. Leonardi-bee J, Jere ml, Britton J. Exposure to parental and sibling smoking and the risk of Smoking uptake in childhood and adolescence: a systematic review and meta-analysis.
45. Gilman Se, Rende R, Boergers J, et al. Parental smoking and adolescent

smoking initiation: an Intergenerational perspective on tobacco control. Pediatrics 2009 ;123(2) : e274-281.
46. Komly V, Le Tourneur A. Burn out among general medical interns: current situation and outlook in metropolitan France. Thesis in Medicine Grenoble; 2011.

47. Chiriaco J. Consumption of psychoactive substances among medical interns: review of the literature and survey of Parisian interns. Medical thesis: Paris 5; 2005.
48. Hérault J. Consommation de substances psychoactives des internes en médecins, enquête auprès des facultés d'Angers et de Lyon. Medical thesis: Angers; 2012.
49. F. Badri, H. Sajiai, L. Amro. Prevalence of smoking among medical and paramedical staff at the CHU Mohamed VI in Marrakech ; Pan Afr Med J. 2017 ; 26 : 45.

50. Wirth N, Spinosa A, Bohadana A, Martinet Y. Different forms of smoking: all as harmful as cigarettes. Rev Prat Med Gen 2007 ; 21 : 79-82.

51. Hill C, Laplanche A. Smoking and mortality: epidemiological aspects. BEH 2003; 22-23: 98-100.
52. Darral KG, Figgins JA. Roll-your-own smoke yields: theorical and practical aspects. Tob Control 1998; 7: 168-75.
53. Martinet Y, Wirth N, Bohadana A, Spinosa A. Smoking and smoking cessation: cannabis use may be accompanied by respiratory complications identical to those associated with smoking. tobacco. The year 2004 in pulmonology. Rev Mal Respir 2005; 22: 5S33- 41.
54. Béatrice Bizet. "De la liberté de fumer en institution", Gérontologie et société 2003/2 (vol. 26 / no. 105), pp. 177-182. DOI 10.3917/gs.105.0177.
55. Perriot J, Llorca PM, Boussiron D, Schwan R. Tabacologie et sevrage tabagique. Paris: John Libbey Eurotext, 2003.
56. Aubin HJ. Nicotine and neuro-psychiatric disorders. Paris: Masson, 1997.
57. Gillet C. Why should alcohol specialists be interested in tobacco? Alcool Addictol 2001 ;23 : 435-605.
58. Collective expertise. Tabac comprendre la dépendance pour agir. Paris Editions INSERM, 2004.
59. Perriot J. Smoking behaviour. Dependance 1996; 8: 23-8.

60. Lebargy F, Becquart LA, Picavet B. Épidémiologie du tabagisme ; Aide à

l'arrêt du tabac. Encycl Med Chir (Elsevier, Paris) AKOS Encyclopédie Pratique de Médecine, 6-0935, 2005, 14 p.
61. Le Houezec J. Nicotine: Abused substance and therapeutic agent. J Psychiatry Neurosci 1998: 23: 95-108.
62. Berlin I, Anthenelli RM. Mono amine oxidases and tobacco smo-king. Int J Neuropsychopharmacol 2001; 4: 33-42.
63. Koob GF, Le Moal M. Drug abuse : hedonic homeostatic dysregulation. Science 1997 ; 278 : 52-8.
64. Koob GF, le Moal M. Drug addiction, dysregulation of reward, and allostasis. Neuropsychopharmacology 2001; 24: 97-124.
65. Jean-Charles Deybach, Delia Cozzolino. Free distribution of nicotine substitutes and smoking cessation. A 3-year observation at the Louis Mourier Hospital. 2008.
66. Tessier Jf, Freour P, Crofton J. French medical students and smoking. Rev Mal Respir 1988 ;589-92.
67. Tessier Jf, Freour P, Nejjari C, Belougne D, Grofton J. Smoking behaviour attitudes of medical students towards smo- king and antismoking comparison : A survey in 10 africans and middle-eastern countries Tobacco Control, 1992 ;95-101.
68. Tessier Jf, Freour P. Smoking habits and attitudes of medical students toward smoking and antismoking compaigns in 9 asian countries. Int J Epidemiol 1992 ;298-304.
69. Rodney Mc: Cigarette smoking among medical students. Am J Public Health 1980 ;70 :169-71.
70. Doll R, Hill A. A study of the aetiology of carcinoma of the lung. Br Med J 1950;19-20:210-3.
71. Peto R, Darby S, Deo H, Silcoks P, Whitley E, Doll R. Smoking, smoking cessation, and lung cancer in the UK since 1950: combination of national statistics with two case-control studies. BMJ 2000;321:323-9.
72. Simonato L, Agudo A, Ahrens W, Benhamou E, Benhamou S, Boffetta P, et al. Lung cancer and cigarette smoking in Europe: an update of risk estimates and an assessment of inter-country heterogeneity. Int J Cancer 2001;91:876-87.
73. Jemal A, Thun MJ, Ries LA, Howe HL, Weir HK, Center MM, et al. Annual report to the nation on the status of cancer, 1975- 2005, featuring trends in lung cancer, tobacco use, and tobacco control. J Natl Cancer Inst 2008;100:1672-94.
74. Ezzati M, Henley SJ, Thun MJ, Lopez AD. Role of smoking in global and

regional cardiovascular mortality. Circulation 2005;112:489-97.
75. Marques-Vidal P, Cambou JP, Ferrières J et al. Distribution and management of cardiovascular risk factors in coronary patients: PREVENIR study. Arch Mal Cœur 2001;94:673-80.
76. Bjartveit K, Tverdal A. Health consequences of smoking 1-4 cigarettes per day. Tob Control 2005;14:315-20.
77. Thomas D. Passive smoking: an essentially cardiovascular impact. La Lettre du Cardiologue 2007;406: 18-22.
78. Wilson K, Gibson N, Willan A, Cook D. Effect of smoking cessation on mortality after myocardial infarction. Metaanalysis of cohort studies. Arch Intern Med 2000;160: 939-44.
79. Critchley JA, Capwell S. Mortality risk reduction associated with smoking cessation in patients with coronary heart disease. A systematic review. JAMA 2003;290:86-97.
80. Yusuf S, Hawken S, Ônpnuu S on behalf of the INTERHEART study investigators. Effect of potentially modifiable risk factors associated with myocardial infarction in 52 countries (the INTERHEART study): a case- control study. Lancet 2004;364:937-5.
81. Teo KK, Ounpuu S, Hawken S, on behalf of the INTERHEART study investigators. Tobacco use and risk of myocardial infarction in 52 countries in the INTERHEART study: a case-control study. Lancet 2006;368:647-58.
82. Canadian Cancer Society (2011). Risk factors for oral cancer. Canadian Cancer Encyclopedia. Retrieved June 16.
83. Cullen, J.W., Blot, W., Henningfield, J., Boyd, G., Mecklenburg, R., and Massey, M.M. (1986 July-August). Health Consequences of Using Smokeless Tobacco: Summary of the Advisory Committee's Report to the Surgeon General. Public Health Reports, 101,355-373.
84. Centres for Disease Control and Prevention. (2004). Smoking and Tobacco Use: 2004 Surgeon General's Report. Retrieved March 2011
85. Neville, B. W. and Day, T. A. (2002), Oral Cancer and Precancerous Lesions. CA: A Cancer Journal for Clinicians, 52,195-215. doi: 10.3322/canjclin.52.4.195.
86. American Dental Association. (1995-2011). Oral Health Topics: Smoking and Tobacco Cessation. Retrieved March 28, 2011.
87. Willigendael EM, Teijink JA, Bartelink M-LL, Peters RJ, Büller HR, Prins MH. Smoking and the patency of lower extremity.
88. Neumayer L, Hosokawa P, Itani K, El-Tamer M, Henderson W, Khuri S. Multivariable Predictors of Postoperative Surgical Site infection after General

and Vascular Surgery: Results from the Patient Safety in Surgery Study. J Am Coll Surg 2007;204:11781187.

89. Campbell D, Henderson W, Englesbe M, Hall B, O'Reilly M, Bratzler D, et al. Surgical site infection prevention: the importance of operative duration and blood transfusion--results of the first American College of Surgeons-National Surgical Quality improvement Program Best Practices Initiative. J Am Coll Surg 2008;207:810-20.

90. Turan A, Mascha EJ, Roberman D, Turner PL, You J, Kurz A, et al.Smoking and perioperative outcomes. Anesthesiology 2011;114:837–46.

91. Hawn M, Houston T, Campagna E, Graham L, Singh J, Bishop M, et al. The Attributable Risk of Smoking on Surgical Complications. Ann Surg 2011;254:914-20.

92. Jones R, Nyawo B, Jamieson S, Clark S. Current smoking predicts increased operative mortality and morbidity after cardiac surgery in the elderly. Interact Cardiovasc Thorac Surg 2011;12:449-53.

93. Mason DP, Subramanian S, Nowicki ER, Grab JD, Murthy SC, Rice TW, et al. Impact of smoking cessation before resection of lung cancer: a Society of Thoracic Surgeons General Thoracic Surgery Database study. Ann Thorac Surg 2009;88:362-70;discussion 370-1.

94. Mills E, Eyawo O, Lockhart I, Kelly S, Wu P, Ebbert J. Smoking cessation reduces postoperative complications: a systematic review and meta-analysis. Am J Med 2011;124:144154.e8.

95. Sørensen L. Wound Healing and Infection in Surgery: The Clinical Impact of Smoking and Smoking Cessation: A Systematic Review and Meta-analysis. Arch Surg 2012;147:373-83.

96. Lassig A, Yueh B, Joseph A. The effect of smoking on perioperative complications in head and neck oncologic surgery. The Laryngoscope 2012;122:1800-1808.

97. Musallam K, Rosendaal F, Zaatari G, Soweid A, Hoballah J, Sfeir P, et al. Smoking and the Risk of Mortality and Vascular and Respiratory Events in Patients Undergoing Major Surgery. JAMA Surgery 2013.

98. Saxena A, Shan L, Reid C, Dinh D, Smith J, Shardey G, et al. Impact of smoking status on early and late outcomes after isolated coronary artery bypass graft surgery. J Cardiol 2013;61.

99. Grønkjær M, Eliasen M, Skov-Ettrup LS, Tolstrup JS, Christiansen AH, Mikkelsen SS, et al. Preoperative smoking status and postoperative complications: a systematic review and meta-analysis. Ann Surg 2014;259:52-

71.
100. Selvarajah S, Black J, Malas M, Lum Y, Propper B, Abularrage C. Preoperative smoking is associated with early graft failure after infrainguinal bypass surgery. J Vasc Surg 2014;59:1308-14.
101. Scolaro J, Schenker M, Yannascoli S, Baldwin K, Mehta S, Ahn J. Cigarette smoking increases complications following fracture: a systematic review. J Bone Joint Surg Am 2014;96:674-81.
102. Pluvy, Panouillères, Garrido, Pauchot, Saboye, Chavoin, et al. Smoking and plastic surgery, part II. Clinical implications: a systematic review with meta-analysis. Ann Chir Plast Esth 2014;60:e15e49.
103. Teng S, Yi C, Krettek C, Jagodzinski M. Smoking and risk of prosthesis-related complications after total hip arthroplasty: a meta- analysis of cohort studies. PLoS ONE 2015;10:e0125294.
104. Imhoff L van, Kranenburg G, Macco S, Nijman N, Overbeeke E van, Wegner I, et al. The prognostic value of continued smoking on survival and recurrence rates in head and neck cancer patients: A systematic review. Head Neck 2015 doi:10.1002/hed.24082.
105. Sriha Belguith A, Elmhamdi S, Bouanene I, Harizi C, Ben Salah A, Ben Salem K, Soltani Essoussi M. Smoking cessation attitudes among adult smokers. Tunis Med. 2015 Mar;93(3):142-7.
106. Hyland A, Borland R, Li Q, Yong HH, McNeill A, Fong GT, et al. Individual level predictors of cessation behaviours among participants in the International Tobacco Control (ITC) Four Country Survey. Tob Control. 2006; 15:83-94.
107. Li L, Borland R, Yong HH, Fong GT, Bansal-Travers M, Quah AC, et al. Predictors of smoking cessation among adult smokers in Malaysia and Thailand: findings from the International Tobacco Control Southeast Asia Survey. Nicotine Tob Res. 2010;12:4-44.
108. Leonardi-bee J, Jere ml, Britton J. Exposure to parental and sibling smoking and the risk of Smoking uptake in childhood and adolescence: a systematic review and meta-analysis.
109. Sienkiewicz-Jarosz H, Zatorski P, Baranowska A, Ryglewicz D, Bienkowski P. Predictors of smoking abstinence after first-ever ischemic stroke: a 3-month follow-up. Stroke. 2009;40 :2592-3.
110. Schiller JS, Ni H. Cigarette smoking and smoking cessation among persons with chronic obstructive pulmonary disease. Am J Health Promot. 2006;20:319-23.

111. Martinson BC, O'Connor PJ, Pronk NP, Rolnick SJ. Smoking cessation attempts in relation to prior health care charges: the effect of antecedent smoking-related symptoms? Am J Health Promot. 2003;18:125-32.
112. Mak YW, Loke AY, Abdullah AS, Lam TH. Household smoking practices of parents with young children, and predictors of poor household smoking practices. Public Health. 2008; 122:1199-209.
113. Ortendahl M. Predicting lapse when stopping smoking among pregnant and non-pregnant women. J Obstet Gynaecol. 2007; 27:138-43.
114. Nollen NL, Mayo MS, Sanderson Cox L, Okuyemi KS, Choi WS, Kaur H, et al. Predictors of quitting among African American light smokers enrolled in a randomized, placebo-controlled trial. J Gen Intern Med. 2006;21:590-5.
115. Oncken C, McKee S, Krishnan-Sarin S, O'Malley S, Mazure CM. Knowledge and perceived risk of smoking-related conditions: a survey of cigarette smokers. Prev Med. 2005;40:779-84.
116. Fidler JA, Shahab L, West R. Strength of urges to smoke as a measure of severity of cigarette dependence: comparison with the Fagerstrom Test for Nicotine Dependence and its components. Addiction. 2011;106:631- 8.
117. Lagrue G, Mautrait C, Béhar C, Cormier S. Development of addictions in adolescents. Role of psychological vulnerability. Alcoologie et addictologie 2005;27 :47-51.
118. Saoussen Bacha, Wissal Skandagi, Mouna Khemiri, Soumaya Oueslati, Naouel Chaouch, Hager Racil, Sana Cheikhrouhou, Mohamed Lamine Megdiche, Abdellatif Chabbou. Evaluation du comportement alimentaire au cours du sevrage tabagique ; La tunisie Medicale - 2016 ; Vol 94 (n°05) : 406-411.
119. Saoussen Bacha, Wissal Skandagi, Mouna Khemiri, Soumaya Oueslati, Naouel Chaouch, Hager Racil, Sana Cheikhrouhou, Mohamed Lamine Megdiche, Abdellatif Chabbou. Evaluation du comportement alimentaire au cours du sevrage tabagique ; La tunisie Medicale - 2016 ; Vol 94 (n°05) : 406-411.Béatrice Bizet. "De la liberté de fumer en institution ", Gérontologie et société 2003/2 (vol. 26 / n° 105),p. 177-182. DOI 10.3917/gs.105.0177.

120. Wirth N, Spinosa A, Bohadana A, Martinet Y. Different forms of smoking: all as harmful as cigarettes. Rev Prat Med Gen 2007; 21 : 79-82.
121. Hill C, Laplanche A. Smoking and mortality: epidemiological aspects. BEH 2003; 22-23: 98-100.
122. Darral KG, Figgins JA. Roll-your-own smoke yields: theorical and practical aspects. Tob Control 1998; 7: 168-75.

123. Martinet Y, Wirth N, Bohadana A, Spinosa A. Smoking and smoking cessation: cannabis use may be accompanied by respiratory complications identical to those associated with tobacco use. L'année 2004 en pneumologie. Rev Mal Respir 2005; 22: 5S33- 41.

APPENDICES

Appendix 1: Questionnaire.

This smoking survey is designed to assess the attitudes and behaviour of medical residents with regard to smoking. Your answers are confidential.

IDENTIFICATION

1. Nationality:□Tunisian□Other (specify):

2. Age years

3. Sex:□masculine □Female

4. You are:□ single□married □other :

5. Before undertake your studies medical studies, where did you live? :

PROFESSIONAL ACTIVITIES

6. You are a : □ **1st year** resident□ **4th** year resident

□ Resident **2nd** year □ Resident **5th** year

□ **3rd** year resident

7. Speciality:

8. Number hours of work per day(excluding excluding day) :

9. Number of shifts per month:

SMOKING :

10. Are you: □smoker□ex-smoker □non-smoker

Depending on whether you are a smoker, ex-smoker or non-smoker, you will answer Part I, II or III.

If you smoke, please complete this section:

11. What type of tobacco do you use?

□Cigarette: number of packs/day:

Number of years smoked : years.

□Pipe□Cigar□Neffa □Chicha: number of times/day:

12. What type of do you smoke?

13. A what age did you smoked your first cigarette?

Years

14. At what age did you start smoking regularly?Years old
15. Level of study at that time□Collège □Lycée □PCEM □DCEM□internat

□ residency

16. Smoking by family and friends: □Father□Mother □Siblings □ Partner

17. How many of cigarettes do you smoke every day?cigarettes/d

18. When do you smoke your first cigarette after waking up?

□Within the first 5 minutes □Between 6 and 30 minutes

□Between 31 and 60 minutes □After 60 minutes

19. Which cigarette do you find indispensable:□ the first□ other □. Please specify:
20. Do you ever smoke when you are ill: no □yes □

21. Do you find it difficult not to smoke in prohibited areas: yes □ no □
22. Main place of smoking: □At homeyou□Ahospital □Other: (Specify
23. Do you smoke more in the morning than in the afternoon? yes □ no □
24. Do you smoke in front of your patients: yes□no □

25. What prompted you to become a smoker? □Stress □Pleasure

□Surroundings

□Better go to concentrate□By user-friendliness □To not not get fat

□Other (specify)

26. What motivates you to continue smoking? □Pleasure Craving □Need □Stimulating effect
□ The habit□Fear of catch of weight gain □Other (Specify):

27. As well as tobacco, do you use any other substances:□Alcohol□cannabis

□ psychotropic drugs□Heroin□amphetamine□cocaine□Other :

28. Has preparing for the residency competition affected your consumption?
□Increase□No change □Decrease

29. Has your period as a boarder affected your consumption?

□Increase □No change□Decrease

30. Do you think your smoking increased during medical school? □Yes □No
31. If yes, on what occasion? □ During examination periods □ During on-call duty □ Other:
32. During your future professional career, do you intend to warn your patients about the risks associated with smoking: □ In the event of smoking-related symptoms or pathologies□ Systematically □ If requested by the patient □ No
33. What do you think your chances are of giving up smoking?

0 10 20 30 40 50 60 70 80 90 100
Aucune chance Toutes les chances

34. Do you think that in 6 months :

□Will you still smoke that much?

□Will you have reduced your cigarette consumption a little?

□Will you have significantly reduced your cigarette consumption?

□Will you have given up smoking?

35. Do you think that in 4 weeks :

□Will you still smoke that much?

□Will you have reduced your cigarette consumption a little?

□Will you have significantly reduced your cigarette consumption?

□Will you have given up smoking?

36. Do you currently want to stop smoking?

Not at all □ A lot □ A lot □

37. Are you ever unhappy about smoking?

Never □Sometimes □Often □Very often □

38. Have you ever tried to stop smoking cigarettes?□Yes□no

39. Number of stop attempts

40. Duration maximum of success of each attempt:
41. What treatment(s) have you used? □ Nicotine substitutes (patches)□

Antidepressants□ Other: (specify)

42. Do you currently feel the urge to stop smoking?□Yes □No

43. If yes, why would you stop smoking?
□ Knowledge of tobacco-related diseases □ Economic reasons

□ To set an example (future doctor) □ Annoyance to family and friends □ Pregnancy□Other :

44. Over the last 2 years, has your tobacco consumption been influenced by the increase in the price of tobacco?
□oui□ no

45. What is the price of a packet of cigarettes that would make you decide to to stop the smoking without hesitation: (in dinars)

46. If nicotine replacement treatments (patch, gum, etc.) or other treatments (antidepressants, etc.) were reimbursed, would this motivate you in your decision to stop smoking? □Yes □No
47. For each of the following diseases, how important a role do you think smoking plays?
- Bladder cancer: □determinant □unrelated □don't know
- coronary artery disease:□determinant □unrelated □don't know
- bronchial cancer : □determinant □unrelated □don't know
- COPD:□determinant□unrelated□don't know
- arteritis:□determinant □unrelated □don't know
- laryngeal cancer: □determinant □unrelated□don't know
- lip-mouth leukoplakia: □determinant □unrelated □don't know

48. In your opinion, is it the doctor's responsibility to convince people to stop smoking?
□strongly agree □not agree □strongly disagree

49. In your opinion, should doctors set a good example by not smoking?
□strongly agree□indifferent□strongly disagree
50. Do you have the knowledge to advise patients who want to stop smoking : □Yes□No
51. Should tobacco advertising be banned completely: □yes □no

52. Should smoking be banned in enclosed public places?

□yes□no

53. Should there be an outright ban on smoking in hospitals?

□yes□no

54. Should healthcare staff be trained to help people who want to stop smoking?
□ yes□noThank you for **your cooperation**
If you are an ex-smoker, please complete this section:

55. Have you ever smoked (daily for 30 days or more without quitting?
□Yes□No
56. Tick the answer that best describes your current situation:

□I have not smoked for less than 6 months

□I haven't smoked in over 6 months

57. A what age did you started à smoking regularly :. years

Your level of education à this time

58. A what age did you stopped from smoking descigarettes :years

Your levelof education à this time

59. How many cigarettes did you smoke each day? cigarettes/d
60. Main place of smoking: □ At home□ In hospital□Other:

61. What prompted you to smoke?□Stress □Pleasure□ People around you

□Other: (Specify)

62. After how many unsuccessful attempts did you make to stop smoking? :
63. Which treatment(s) have you used?□Nicotine substitutes (patches)
□Other:

64. Do you think your smoking has increased during your medical studies?
□ Yes□ No

65. If yes, on what occasion?□ During examination periods □ During on-call duty □Other:

66. Why did you stop smoking?

□ Tobacco-related diseases□ Economic reasons

□ Pressure from family and friends□To set an example (futuredoctor)
□Pregnancy □Health problems

Other:(please specify)

67. Do you currently feel an urge to become a smoker again?□ Yes□ No
68. Smoking in close circle: □ Father □ Mother □ Brother(s) and sister(s) □ Partner

69. During your future professional career, do you intend to warn your patients about the risks associated with smoking?
□ Systematically

□ If requested by the patient

□ In the event of symptoms or pathologies linked to smoking

70. For each of the following diseases, how important a role do you think smoking plays?
- Bladder cancer: □determinant □unrelated □don't know
- coronary artery disease:□determinant □unrelated □don't know
- bronchial cancer : □determinant □unrelated □don't know
- COPD:□determinant□unrelated□don't know
- arteritis:□determinant □unrelated □don't know
- laryngeal cancer: □determinant □unrelated□don't know
- lip-mouth leukoplakia: □determinant □unrelated □don't know

71. In your opinion, is it the doctor's responsibility to convince people to stop smoking?
□strongly agree □not agree □strongly disagree

72. In your opinion, should doctors set a good example by not smoking?
□strongly agree□indifferent□strongly disagree

73. Do you have the knowledge to advise patients who want to stop smoking : □Yes□No
74. Should tobacco advertising be banned completely: □yes□no

75. Should smoking be banned in enclosed public places?

□ yes□no

76. Should there be an outright ban on smoking in hospitals?

□ yes□no

77. Should healthcare staff be trained to help people who want to stop smoking? □yes□no

Thank you for your cooperation
If you are a non-smoker, please complete this section:

78. Have you tried cigarettes at least once: □not□in childhood□during medical studies
79. Do you know anyone who smokes: □ Father □ Mother □ Brother(s) and sister(s) □ Partner
80. Do you feel like smoking? □non□sometimes□always

81. Where do you feel you are most exposed to other people's smoking?

□At you□A Hospital □Other

82. For each of the following diseases, how important a role do you think smoking plays?

- Bladder cancer: □determinant □unrelated □don't know
- coronary artery disease:□determinant □unrelated □don't know
- bronchial cancer : □determinant □unrelated □don't know
- COPD:□determinant□unrelated□don't know
- arteritis:□determinant □unrelated □don't know
- laryngeal cancer: □determinant □unrelated□don't know
- lip-mouth leukoplakia: □determinant □unrelated □don't know

83. In your opinion, is it the doctor's responsibility to convince people to stop smoking?
□strongly agree □not agree □strongly disagree

84. In your opinion, should doctors set a good example by not smoking?
□strongly agree □not agree □strongly disagree

85. Do you have the knowledge to advise patients who want to stop smoking: □Yes□No
86. Should tobacco advertising be banned completely: □yes□no
87. Should smoking be banned in enclosed public places?

□ yes□no

88. Should there be an outright ban on smoking in hospitals?

□ yes□no

89. Should healthcare staff be trained to help people who want to stop smoking? □yes□no
90. Why do you think some doctors smoke? □ Pleasure □ Craving

□The stimulating effect

□Need □ Habit□ Fear of weight gain □ Other (Specify):

91. What situations do you think might prompt a doctor to stop smoking?
□ Tobacco-related diseases□ Economic reasons

□ Pressure from family and friends□To set an example (futuredoctor)
□Pregnancy□ Health problems

□ Other:(please specify)

Thank you for your cooperation

Appendix 2: Fagerström test

How soon after waking up do you smoke your first cigarette?
Within five minutes (3)
From 6 to 30 minutes (2)
From 31 to 60 minutes (1)
More than 60 minutes (0)
Do you find it difficult to refrain from smoking in places where it is prohibited?
Yes (1)
No (0)
Which cigarette of the day would be the hardest for you to give up?
The first (1)
Any other (0)
How many cigarettes do you smoke a day?
10 or less (0)
From 11 to 20 (1)
From 21 to 30 (2)
31 or more (3)
Do you smoke more in the morning than in the afternoon?
Yes (1)
No (0)
Do you smoke even when you're so ill you have to stay in bed most of the day?
Yes (1)
No (0)
Result:
2 points: no nicotine dependence
4 points: low nicotine dependence
6 points: average nicotine dependence
8 points: high nicotine dependence
10 points: very high nicotine dependence.

SUMMARY

Issues :
Smoking is a real public health problem. Medical residents are a socio-professional category concerned by the subject of tobacco, both its consumption and patients' attitudes to smoking.

Goals :
To study the epidemiological factors of smoking among residents, their smoking habits and the practice of minimal smoking cessation advice for their patients.

Methods :
We carried out a cross-sectional frequency calculation: prevalence study on 285 medical residents working at the Hedi Chaker and Habib Bourguiba University Hospitals in Sfax during the first half of 2016.

Results :
The total number of residents in the Sfax university hospitals during the study period was 285, with an overall participation rate of 77.98%. The highest percentage of residents surveyed was female (52.70%). The majority of residents surveyed lived in Sfax (92.8%). The participating residents had medical specialties (123 residents), surgical specialties (60 residents) and basic specialties (36 residents). The prevalence of smoking among residents was 32.88%. The group of smokers is represented by 73 residents, 97.26% of whom are male. The age group most affected was between 27 and 29. The majority of residents who smoked were in surgical specialties, with a prevalence of 73.33%. The majority of residents reported an increase in smoking during their internship and residency. Several factors were predictive of smoking initiation. The most common was stress (49.3%), followed by pleasure (19.2%). Craving was the most common predictor of continued smoking, accounting for 32.88%. Only 8.22% of residents who smoked had a strong desire to stop smoking at the time of the survey. We noted that 158 residents were prepared to provide their patients with minimal advice systematically, i.e. 71.70% of all residents surveyed. We noted that 86.3% of residents who smoked thought they had sufficient knowledge to convince patients who wanted to stop smoking. It was noted that 29 residents had tried to quit at least once. Of the 29 residents who wanted to give up smoking, 24 attributed this to their knowledge of tobacco-

related illnesses. The majority of residents were in favour of banning tobacco advertising and its use in public places and hospitals. All the residents were in favour of training medical and paramedical staff to help them stop smoking.

Conclusion:

Smoking is a major public health problem. Medical residents represent a socio-professional category concerned by this problem in two main ways: their smoking habits and their knowledge of the harmful effects of smoking, as well as their involvement in the fight against smoking, helping people to stop smoking and providing medical advice to their patients.

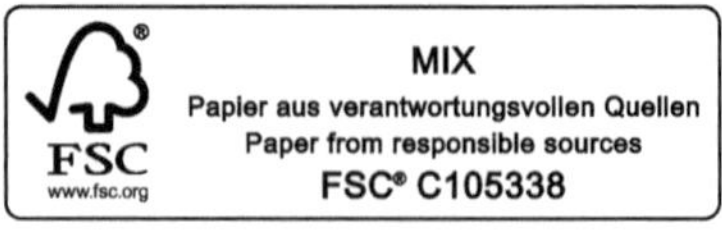

Printed by Books on Demand GmbH, Norderstedt / Germany